D0792125

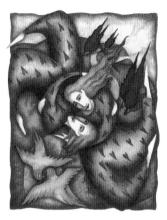

HEALTH AND HEALING
THE NATURAL WAY

STAY HAPPY,
STAY WELL

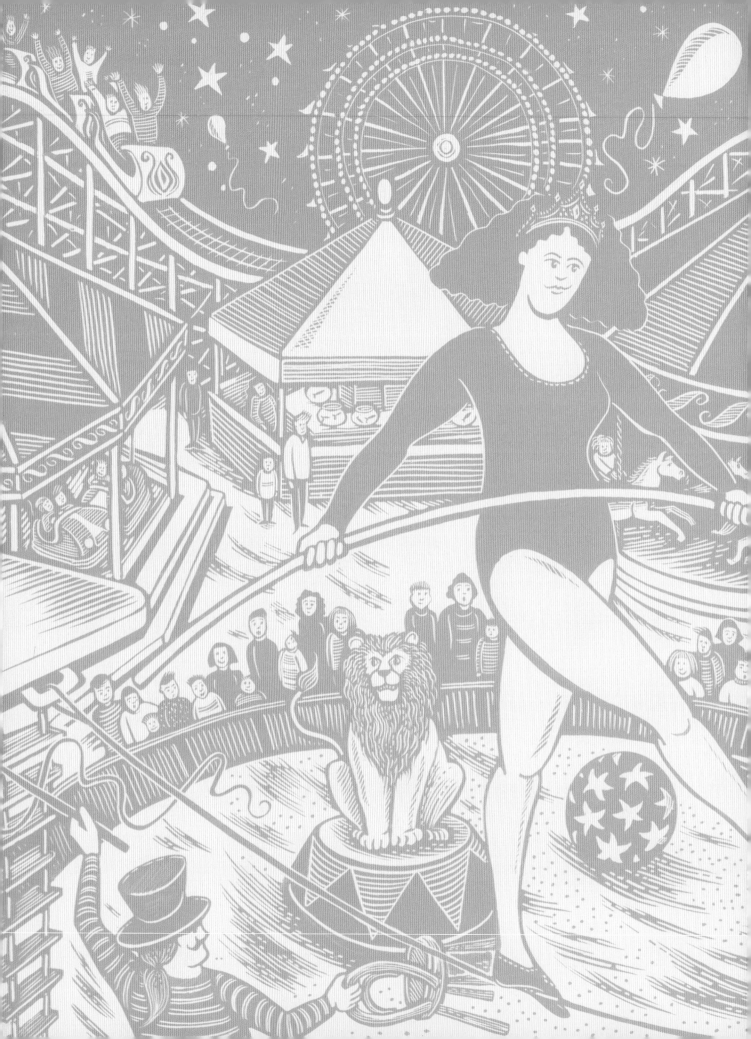

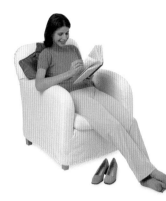

*HEALTH AND HEALING
THE NATURAL WAY*

STAY HAPPY,
STAY WELL

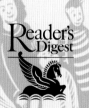

Reader's
Digest

PUBLISHED BY

THE READER'S DIGEST ASSOCIATION LIMITED

LONDON NEW YORK SYDNEY MONTREAL CAPE TOWN

A READERS DIGEST BOOK
produced by
Carroll & Brown Limited, London

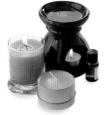

CARROLL & BROWN

Publishing Director Denis Kennedy
Art Director Chrissie Lloyd

Managing Editor Sandra Rigby
Managing Art Editor Tracy Timson

Project Coordinator Laura Price

Editor Angela Newton

Art Editor Simon Daley
Designer Evie Loizides

Photographers David Murray, Jules Selmes

Production Karen Kloot, Wendy Rogers

Computer Management John Clifford, Paul Stradling

Copyright © 2000 The Reader's Digest Association, Inc.
Copyright © 2000 The Reader's Digest Association (Canada) Ltd.
Copyright © 2000 Reader's Digest Association Far East Ltd.
Philippine Copyright © 2000 Reader's Digest Association Far East Ltd.

All rights reserved. Unauthorized reproduction,
in any manner, is prohibited.

® Reader's Digest and the Pegasus logo are
registered trademarks of The Reader's Digest Association, Inc.

Printed in the United States of America

Library of Congress Cataloging in Publication Data

Stay happy, stay well
    p. cm. — (Health and healing the natural way)
Includes index
ISBN 0-7621-0281-0
    1. Health. 2. Health—Psychological aspects
3. Mind and body. 4. Happiness.
I. Reader's Digest Association. II. Series.

RA776.5 .S757 2000
613—dc21
                                                00-020387

Address any comments about *Stay Happy, Stay Well* to
Editor in Chief, U.S. Illustrated Reference Books,
Pleasantville, NY 10570

CONSULTANTS

David M. Warburton BSc, AM, PhD,
CPsychol, FPsSOC, FRSA
Professor of Psychopharmacology, University of Reading
Janice Rigby BA (Hons) M. Psychol, Dip. CBT
Chartered clinical psychologist
Kharmabunda BA (Hons)
Centre Director at The London Buddhist Centre

CONTRIBUTORS

Susan Conder BA, MA, Dip. Psychodynamic
Marital & Couple Counselling
Marriage guidance counsellor
Victoria Davenport
Psychoanalytic psychotherapist
Patrick McGhee MA, DPhil, CPsychol, AFBPsS, FRSA
Chartered psychologist
Peter L.N. Naish BSc, DPhil, CPsychol,
AFBPsS, MBSECH
*University lecturer, hypnotist, and principal psychologist
at The Centre for Human Sciences*

WRITER

Ian Wood

READER'S DIGEST PROJECT STAFF

Series Editor Gayla Visalli
Editorial Director, Health & Medicine Wayne Kalyn
Design Director Barbara Rietschel
Production Technology Manager Douglas A. Croll
Editorial Manager Christine R. Guido
Art Production Coordinator Jennifer R. Tokarski

READER'S DIGEST ILLUSTRATED REFERENCE BOOKS, U.S.

Editor in Chief Christopher Cavanagh
Art Director Joan Mazzeo
Operations Manager William J. Cassidy

The information in this book is for reference only;
it is not intended as a substitute for a doctor's diagnosis and care.
The editors urge anyone with continuing medical problems
or symptoms to consult a doctor.

STAY HAPPY, STAY WELL

More and more people today are choosing to take greater responsibility for their own health care rather than relying on a doctor to step in with a cure when something goes wrong. We now recognize that we can influence our health by making improvements in lifestyle, for example, eating better, getting more exercise, and reducing stress. People are also becoming increasingly aware that there are other healing methods—some of them new, others ancient—that can help prevent illness or be used as a complement to orthodox medicine.

The series *Health and Healing the Natural Way* will help you to make your own health choices by giving you clear, comprehensive, straightforward, and encouraging information and advice about methods of improving your health. The series explains the many different natural therapies that are now available, including aromatherapy, herbalism, acupressure, and a number of others, and the circumstances in which they may be of benefit when used in conjunction with conventional medicine.

STAY HAPPY, STAY WELL examines the influence that our thoughts, emotions, and attitudes can have on our general well-being and on how we live our lives. It explains how being honest with yourself about your real feelings and learning to challenge negative thought patterns can enable you to live life to your full potential. The book also provides practical advice on how to improve both your emotional and physical health and outlines self-help strategies for developing self-awareness and promoting relaxation. It describes some common mental problems, including depression, phobias, and addictions, plus various conventional and complementary treatment options for them. Taking into account biological, psychological, and cultural factors, *STAY HAPPY, STAY WELL* shows you how to develop and maintain a positive outlook and achieve a sense of balance and vitality.

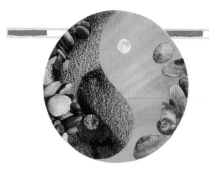

CONTENTS

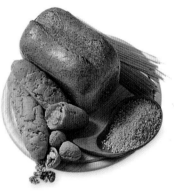

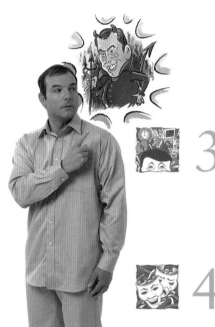

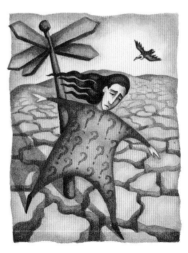

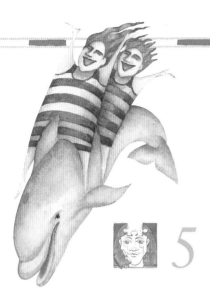

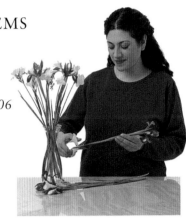

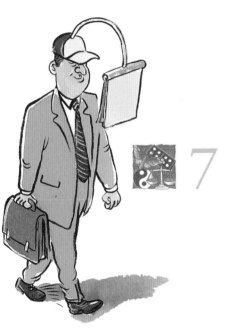

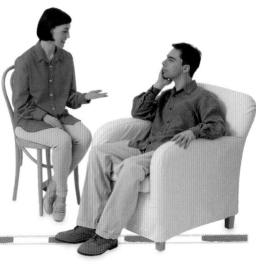

THE MIND-BODY CONNECTION

Increasingly, scientific evidence is emerging to prove that our thoughts and emotions can have a profound influence on our health and well-being.

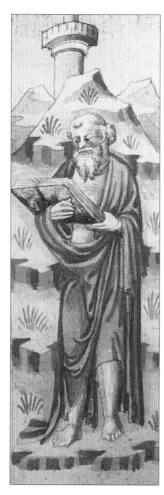

EPICURUS
The Greek philosopher set up a commune in Athens where members could live in peaceful friendship.

The nature of the link between mind and body and the relative influence of one over the other have been discussed by philosophers and physicians for centuries. Both Eastern and Western traditions have asserted that for people to be physically well, they must also be mentally and emotionally healthy. The ancient Greek philosopher Epicurus taught that pleasure is the natural aim of all humankind and, when achieved, can lead to freedom from debilitating pain and the effects of anxiety. He established a school of philosophy known as the Gardens, where people could live in peaceful friendship and tranquillity, seeking health and happiness in simple, honorable lives.

The teachings of Epicurus have been distorted through the dark glass of history. Today Epicureanism is associated with sensual, hedonistic pleasures, and the crux of the philosopher's teachings is ignored. Nevertheless, the beliefs of Epicurus have remained in the forefront of much medical practice. The Renaissance physician Paracelsus, for example, emphasized the importance of considering emotions, thoughts, and fears, as well as physical symptoms, when treating a patient. He claimed that a man was a true physician only when he realized the significance of "that which is unnamed, invisible, and immaterial, yet has its effect." Essentially, he believed that a condition of the body could be fully understood only when it was put in the context of a patient's emotional state.

It is worth noting that the very word *disease* suggests a lack of pleasure—or dis-ease. The modern word *ease* comes from the Latin term *ansatus*, which means "elbows in a relaxed state." Disease therefore describes having insufficient elbow room, a sense of discomfort or inhibition of natural pleasure. So the word we now use to describe physical illness etymologically relates to displeasure. Being unwell means being unhappy—essentially, being at odds with how one should normally feel.

THE PHYSICAL LINK

The importance of the mind-body connection is steadily gaining wider acceptance. Doctors are realizing more and more that physical symptoms can be brought on or worsened by such emotional conditions as stress, depression, or suppressed anger. Most people have experienced a cold that never seems to go away or a migraine headache that develops after an extended period of tension. Times of great emotional stress, such as bereavement, marital difficulties, or prolonged pressure at work, have all been associated with physical conditions that range from stomach ulcers to flu to stiff joints.

The low self-esteem that often comes with negative moods can affect a person's ability to recover from a condition or can accentuate its symptoms even further. As frustration at feeling unwell increases, a person may become even more emotionally upset and negative in outlook. This cycle of depression and ill health then affects every aspect of the individual's life, causing lethargy, emotional negativity, and a general sense of futility.

After centuries of philosophical supposition and reliance on circumstantial evidence concerning the physiological link between the health of the body and the mind, the connection has been proved only in recent times. Scientists have now shown that the immune system can be both controlled and disrupted by activity in the brain. Under normal circumstances any foreign invader in the body is either neutralized or destroyed by white blood cells, part of the body's defense system. However, when we experience negative emotions, such as anxiety, or undergo intense pressure for long periods, the brain stimulates the production of certain hormones that interfere with signals sent from the central nervous system to the immune cells, decreasing their ability to function efficiently. Distressed people are therefore more likely to succumb to infections and may take longer to recover from minor illness than people who are emotionally calmer. Studies of people suffering from depression after a traumatic experience show that they tend to have weaker and less efficient immune responses.

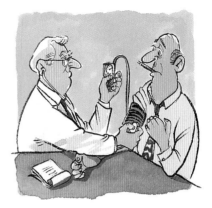

PHYSICAL MANIFESTATIONS
Most people now accept the premise that mental stress and prolonged anxiety can produce physical symptoms, such as raised blood pressure.

THE BODY'S DEFENSES
Lymphocytes, a type of white blood cell shown colored here, help fight off infections and disease. Prolonged stress can inhibit their efficiency.

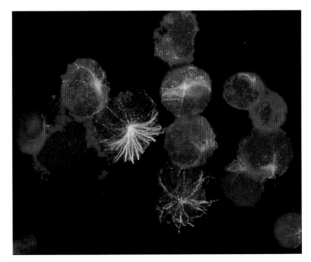

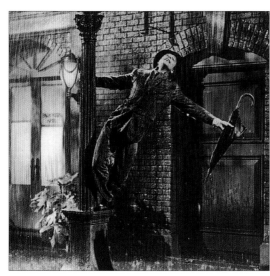

WHAT YOU CAN DO

Medical evidence suggests that the fitter and healthier we are physically, the better we are equipped to cope with emotional crises. At the same time, nurturing a positive mental attitude can improve our chances of enjoying the benefits of an efficient immune system and a physically active and healthy life. Of course, people differ in their physical and mental dispositions, and nobody can help falling ill occasionally or having a bad day now and then. Nevertheless, depending on personality and temperament, some individuals set up a variety of support networks and emotional safety nets that will help them cope in moments of difficulty, and others do not. For example, insular people, who tend to avoid expressing emotion, may suffer from chronic emotional frustration and physical ill health. On the other hand, more assertive persons, who are normally less inhibited about expressing personal feelings, are less likely to suffer from stress-related illness. An outgoing personality and a certain amount of emotional honesty enable these people to pursue the activities and behavior that are conducive to good health.

Experts agree that a healthy, active lifestyle has the potential to make you not only physically fitter but also emotionally healthier. The benefits of exercise in relieving stress have been well documented. Endorphins, which are natural mood-enhancing chemicals, are produced more prolifically during physical exertion and thus help us to feel a natural high after exercising. Studies have also shown that regular exercise combined with a good, balanced diet helps to increase natural energy levels. This can improve your sense of vitality and enthusiasm, making everyday tasks seem easier and helping to limit periods of lethargy and general listlessness.

THE PURSUIT OF HAPPINESS

While the evidence is clear that we are healthiest when we are happy, it is more difficult to determine exactly what does make us happy. The volumes that have been written about utopias and ideal lifestyles are proof that we believe absolute contentment is possible. Across different generations, cultures, and religions, people have always striven to find the secrets of greater

A BALANCED DIET
Simple steps like eating healthy, well-balanced meals will help to improve your resistance to illness.

ETERNAL OPTIMISM
Gene Kelly's rendition of "Singin' in the Rain" embodies the idea of keeping a positive frame of mind.

happiness, firm in the belief that there is some kind of strategy that can improve emotional well-being. While Christianity has often asserted the importance of virtue in constructing happiness, many Eastern traditions teach that happiness is a question of spiritual and physical balance. The Noble Eightfold Path of Buddhism, for example, and the *Tao Te Ching* (the major text) of Taoism advocate the achievement of emotional well-being through both internal balance of the mind, spirit, and body and external harmony with the environment of the natural world and the people around us. They assert that exercise, diet, and attitude of mind are all intrinsic elements in building a sense of complete harmony.

The Buddhist framework of finding an ideal "middle way," a path between extremes, is appropriate for most people, regardless of their religion. In seeking to pursue moderation in all things, it is possible to find a balance both in our internal lives and in our relationship with the world around us. In fact, Buddhists believe that enlightenment, the ultimate human achievement, is reached by avoiding excess in both our physical and emotional lives. Human life is seen as a struggle to maintain equilibrium and find the best options and experiences in every moment.

TAKING CONTROL

Although you cannot control everything that will happen in your life, confidence in your own abilities can help you achieve much of what you desire. There is no one special path to contentment, nor one particular way to become healthier, so STAY HAPPY, STAY WELL examines the many different attitudes, theories, and practical strategies that people have devised to improve mental and physical health. Throughout the book there are visualization exercises that can help to promote relaxation and develop self-awareness. Chapter 1 takes a look at recent evidence that supports the mind-body theory and the numerous influences that have contributed to modern psychological belief. An overview of the many different theories and therapies that have been devised for mental health

PARADISE ON EARTH
The eternal quest for happiness is embodied in the belief in the existence of heaven, which has been brought to earth in mythological and literary accounts of utopias. One such myth is about the island of Atlantis, a "perfect land" that has been described and searched for throughout history. According to legend, Poseidon, the Greek god of the sea, landed on Atlantis, heralded by nymphs and porpoises. He found it so perfect he decided to live there, but Atlantis was eventually swallowed by the sea.

FLOWER POWER
Flowers have long played a part in promoting relaxation and improving emotional health. The wild rose, for example, is used in aromatherapy and Bach flower remedies to help relieve stress.

ALTERNATIVE EXERCISE
Quindo is a relatively new therapy that uses exercises to promote both mental and physical balance.

provides a background for understanding contemporary approaches to treatment of emotional problems.

The experiences and anxieties that contribute to an individual's development are examined in Chapter 2. The formative years of childhood, the occasionally disorienting experience of young adulthood, and the necessary readjustment of advancing age can all affect our perspective on life, bringing change in opportunities, attitudes, and health. Our genetic makeup, combined with social, cultural, and personal influences, helps to determine the kind of person we are and how we cope.

The power and ability of the mind is considered in Chapter 3, which examines how we can direct our thoughts and emotions to achieve the very best in our emotional and physical lives. Some emotions and their effects are examined in greater detail in Chapter 4, which looks at how "bad" as well as "good" emotions are necessary for personal health and how some negative emotions can be channeled in more constructive ways. Emotions that are generally seen as negative, such as guilt or envy, are shown to be normal experiences that need to be acknowledged and controlled in order to gain a sense of completeness.

Chapter 5 looks at some of the more serious illnesses and conditions that can affect a person's mind and perspective. In addition to common phobias and addictions, the chapter examines the damaging cycle of depression and its potential threat to emotional and physical well-being.

Chapter 6 discusses many of the therapies that can be used to counteract serious disorders and improve general outlook. The psychological theories of Sigmund Freud, along with with Eastern and holistic therapies, demonstrate the numerous ways in which therapists can help address specific emotional problems or simply enhance relaxation and encourage emotional honesty.

Finally, Chapter 7 looks at ways in which we can help ourselves to achieve and maintain balance in our lives. Using the evidence for mental and physical connections, it suggests ways in which you can improve your general lifestyle and outlook and maximize your chances of enjoying a life of good health and happiness.

ACHIEVING HEALTH AND HAPPINESS

Believing that you are in control of your own life is one of the secrets to happiness and contentment. It is also important in helping you to maintain a healthy lifestyle. Although no one has the power to control every aspect of life, if you strive to be as emotionally and physically complete as possible, your body will function at its optimum and you will feel happy and fulfilled much of the time.

Q DO YOU CONSTANTLY SUFFER FROM MINOR ILLNESSES?

Although many complaints have a medical cause, there is now little doubt that many symptoms can be caused or made worse by negative emotional states. Chapter 1 looks at how the mind and body can influence each other and affect your health and well-being.

Q DO YOU OFTEN QUESTION YOUR EMOTIONS?

Most people occasionally respond inappropriately to a situation. They get very angry, fall head over heels in love, or feel excessively sad about a minor event. This is perfectly normal, as long as it does not happen too often, and it shows that you are emotionally alert to your environment. Nevertheless, it can be useful to take stock of your situation and consider how common these excessive demonstrations of emotion are. Chapter 4 looks at how all of us sometimes mistakenly expect emotions like love to be a direct link to happiness and how it may benefit us to take a closer look at the way we behave emotionally.

Q DO YOU OFTEN FEEL LOW?

Identifying and addressing a situation that is causing you emotional pain may help you find a way out of an apparently bleak situation. It is important to approach problems from different angles and look at the variety of options that are available to you. A general review of your lifestyle or diet, for example, may help you to refocus your outlook and develop approaches that can help you feel better about yourself. Chapter 7 looks at many of the important steps you can take in terms of exercise, diet, and attitude to reach a better level of both physical and emotional fitness.

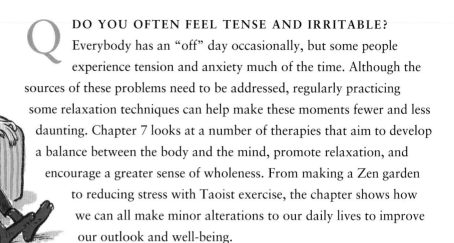

Q DO YOU OFTEN FEEL TENSE AND IRRITABLE?

Everybody has an "off" day occasionally, but some people experience tension and anxiety much of the time. Although the sources of these problems need to be addressed, regularly practicing some relaxation techniques can help make these moments fewer and less daunting. Chapter 7 looks at a number of therapies that aim to develop a balance between the body and the mind, promote relaxation, and encourage a greater sense of wholeness. From making a Zen garden to reducing stress with Taoist exercise, the chapter shows how we can all make minor alterations to our daily lives to improve our outlook and well-being.

Q DO YOU WANT TO LEARN THE SECRET OF POSITIVE THINKING?

Chapter 3 looks at how the mind can affect self-esteem and how positive thinking techniques can help us to see the world and ourselves in a better light. Examining how we receive and process information, the chapter provides some ideas on how to make the most of these processes. It also offers some tips on bettering your self-perception.

Q ARE YOU WORRIED ABOUT MENTAL ILLNESS?

Many people find the terms and definitions used to describe serious psychological disorders bewildering. Chapter 5 explains the differences between mild and chronic depression, the sources of many phobias and addictions, and the actions we can take to minimize the risks of developing mental problems. Chapter 6 investigates the range of therapies, from Freudian psychoanalysis to medications to group therapy, that are available today.

DO YOU KNOW WHAT HAPPINESS MEANS?

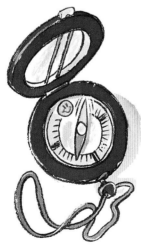

Q Everybody has different expectations, desires, and aspirations in life. There is no one key to happiness, but setting up the right foundations with a fit, healthy body and an open, relaxed mind is a good way to begin. It is important to develop a sense of direction, knowing that even when things occasionally go wrong, you are essentially on the right track. Aspiring to happiness means having a good sense of what you want out of life and setting reasonable targets. Learning to take control and improving your sense of direction could be the first step to greater emotional completeness and real health and happiness.

CHAPTER 1

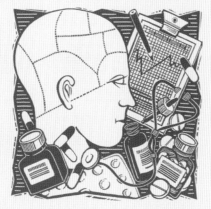

BEING HAPPY, BEING WELL

*Your state of mind can affect your physical
health in powerful ways. Whether you suffer from
constant colds or tension headaches or a more
serious complaint like depression, research
increasingly shows that your outlook can make
a dramatic difference in your general well-being.
But exactly how does this happen and what can
we do to achieve health in mind and body?*

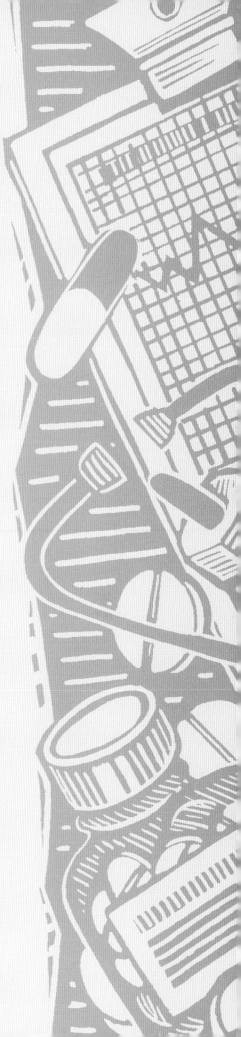

HAPPINESS AND THE IMMUNE SYSTEM

In recent years scientists have proved what many philosophers and physicians have believed for centuries: your thoughts and emotions can play a role in causing and relieving physical illness.

The interplay between the brain and the body is a continual one. As the brain instructs the lungs to breathe and the heart to pump, the body provides fresh supplies of blood and oxygen to the active brain. Similarly, if the body experiences some kind of physical disturbance or pain, it is the brain that interprets these signals and responds by telling the body to react. But if the mind is fatigued or undergoing some kind of emotional pain, this can affect the body in a physical way.

Doctors and psychiatrists are becoming increasingly aware of the mutual influences between the mind and body. Just as constant physical throbbing can lead to mental distress, an emotional problem can influence a physical condition. If a hurt is due to mental or emotional disturbance, this does not mean that the physical symptom is any less real or painful for the person who is experiencing it. We are all familiar with the short-term wave of nausea that can accompany a job interview or a tension headache that can arise from a hectic day at work, but researchers now believe that the mind and emotions affect the body to such an extent that they can influence our long-term health.

THE IMMUNE SYSTEM

Until the mid-1970s the majority of scientists believed that the immune system, which is the fundamental basis of health, functioned independently of the brain and psychological processes. In 1975, however, the psychologist Robert Ader and the immunologist Nicholas Cohen produced a landmark study demonstrating that the immune system was influenced by the brain. They conducted tests in which they gave rats sugar-flavored water containing a drug that suppressed the immune system. When they later gave the rats sugar-flavored water without the drug, the drink still suppressed the rats' immune systems, even though no chemical was present. It appeared that in a complex interplay of brain and body, the animals' immune systems had been conditioned to decline regardless of whether the ingested substance should have that effect.

Subsequent studies have revealed that the central nervous system and the immune system are directly linked. Fibers of the sympathetic nervous system affect virtually every organ of the immune system; in particular they influence the production of lymphocytes, white blood cells in the body that are responsible for protecting us from viruses, bacteria, and tumor cells.

Research has also shown that stress in general affects the immune system. This stress could be the result of an extreme event, such as death or divorce, or stem from more everyday forms of psychological tension, such as boredom, anxiety over work, or frustration.

In 1991 psychologist Sheldon Cohen conducted a study of 400 healthy volunteers to try to establish factors that can predispose people to catching a cold. All the participants were exposed to the same cold virus and then quarantined together in apartments under controlled conditions. Surprisingly, the study found that the most

THE IMPORTANCE OF RELAXATION Research has shown that the immune system works at its optimum when you feel calm and unstressed.

THE EFFECTS OF STRESS ON THE IMMUNE SYSTEM

There is now solid scientific evidence that stress and prolonged anxiety can affect physical health. When we experience intense emotional feelings, the brain stimulates the pituitary gland to release hormones into the bloodstream. These chemicals not only alert the body to stress but also interfere with the hormones of the immune system, weakening its response to disease. One such chemical is cortisol, which inhibits the ability of white blood cells to produce antibodies. Unable to fight off or neutralize foreign invaders efficiently, the body comes under increased risk of contracting ailments and illnesses.

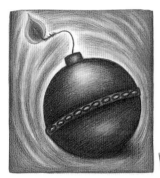

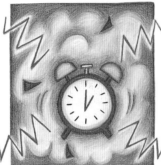

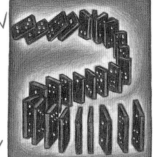

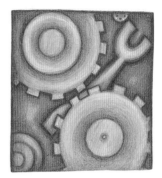

A startling event or moment of distress—experiencing an earthquake or the death of a loved one, for example—causes a significant wave of emotion through the body.

The impulse then activates the pituitary gland to secrete hormones. These chemicals also stimulate reactions in other parts of the body, like the adrenal glands.

The adrenal glands help the body to prepare for "fight or flight," but they also release the chemical cortisol, which disrupts the functioning of white blood cells.

If the body suffers from a prolonged presence of cortisol—as a result of continual stress, for example—the white blood cells will be unable to fight off disease.

significant factor in determining whether the participants caught a cold was their level of stress. Even taking into account such varied factors as age, sex, diet, and level of physical activity, the key contributor seemed to be the amount of psychological stress an individual was experiencing.

The evidence strongly suggests that a healthy emotional state is essential for good physical health. Indeed, the ability of the mind to affect the behavior of the body has been proved repeatedly. Experiments conducted at the University of Oslo, for instance, revealed that the mind can play an intrinsic part in developing illness. A group of young men who were in good health were all informed that they had high blood pressure. Six months later the men recorded far higher pressures than in their previous measurements. It seems that concern and belief in the existence of the condition led to a physical reaction.

THE HOLISTIC APPROACH

Although Western science has only recently started to investigate the link between mind and body, many ancient Eastern philosophies are based on this concept of integration. For example, if you were to visit a doctor of traditional Chinese medicine because you had severe back pain, you would be assessed for physiological symptoms *and* your psychological state in order to determine the appropriate form of treatment. A similar approach is found in the ancient Indian health system of Ayurveda. Both traditions believe that health, happiness, and longevity are based on the harmonious operation of mind, body, and spirit. Ignoring the health of your mind will inevitably lead to health problems for your body and vice versa.

For Eastern practitioners no single aspect of well-being is any more important than another. A balanced diet, exercise, and a relaxed mental state are all integral factors of general good health. This is why Eastern forms of exercise, like yoga, feature deep breathing and relaxation techniques that promote mental calmness, in addition to exercise for the physical body.

In the West we are beginning to embrace these concepts as the widespread benefits of a healthy lifestyle are increasingly understood and acknowledged. For example, exercise and a healthy diet are now recognized as useful means of releasing stress, as well as providing other important health benefits.

BRAIN ACTIVITY
The red area in this PET scan shows the concentration of brain activity around the hypothalamus that occurs when a person experiences fear.

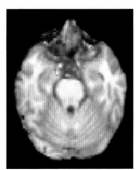

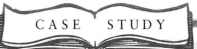

A Constantly Ill Mother

Emotional and mental stress can affect the body's immune system. Prolonged anxiety and tension often find expression in physical symptoms and a general feeling of ill health. If the emotional cause of the problem is not addressed, these symptoms can become a regular feature of your daily life, producing debilitating effects.

Polly is 26 and a single parent of a two-year-old daughter, Rachel. She works as a secretary in a busy law firm but would like a change of career and is now studying part-time for a degree in art history. Ever since she and her husband split up, Polly has found it very difficult to juggle all of her commitments and pay the bills. Most of her weekends and evenings are spent looking after her daughter while trying to study. For the past eight months Polly has been suffering from constant flulike symptoms, and she now feels under greater pressure because of approaching year-end exams. She often feels lightheaded and tired from lack of sleep and poor breathing. Her doctor believes that her symptoms could be stress related.

WHAT SHOULD POLLY DO?

Polly is obviously under great pressure from many angles, and the emotional stress is affecting her immune system, so she is more susceptible to catching colds and other viruses. To improve her health, she must try to relieve at least some of the pressures in her life. Although she feels she cannot call on her ex-husband for help with childcare, she should ask her family or close friends if they can help. This will give her more time for study and relaxation. She also needs to review her financial situation carefully. Finding ways to reduce her expenses and talking to her creditors about lowering her monthly payments until she is able to make more money would ease the burden.

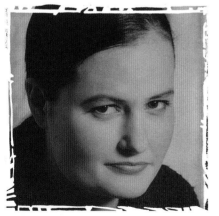

FINANCE
Worrying about money is a prime cause of prolonged stress and tension.

HOME
Juggling a career and a family can be particularly difficult if you are trying to do it on your own.

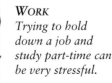

WORK
Trying to hold down a job and study part-time can be very stressful.

Action Plan

HOME
Family commitments need to be prioritized. Getting support for some of the chores will help to relieve pressure.

WORK
Balance work with relaxation to diminish stress. If pressures become too much, think about how to get some practical help.

FINANCES
See a financial counselor about ways to bring spending and bill paying under control. Seek to reduce monthly payments to relieve financial pressure.

HOW THINGS TURNED OUT FOR POLLY

Polly's mother now picks up Rachel from nursery school twice a week and enjoys this special time with her granddaughter. By the time Polly gets home on those evenings, Rachel has already been fed, so Polly has more time to study. Polly was worried that she could not afford her next term's fees but found out she could pay in installments. This has eased the pressures on her a little, and she is feeling better both physically and mentally.

HAPPINESS AND A HEALTHY MIND

Although most people would agree that a positive mental outlook is vital for well-being, it is not easy to define exactly what happiness is or how it might be achieved. For some persons happiness is embodied in the meeting of personal aspirations—a state in which most desires and needs are met and emotional security is untarnished by the worries of everyday life. For instance, many people associate childhood with happiness, as if innocence and freedom from care were essential requirements.

In contrast, many psychological theories and religious philosophies see true contentment linked to a sense of peace and inner calmness. Far from being based on a state of innocence and aspiration, this inner peace has at its root a recognition of the realities of everyday existence. It includes an ability to accept both ourselves and others as we are. The psychological theories of Sigmund Freud and Carl Jung, for example, propose that in order to be truly happy and fully integrated, we must accept all aspects of ourselves. This state involves a release from old anxieties, insecurities, and fears so that we can reach a state of self-confidence and contentment. They suggest that it is only in accepting the realities of everyday existence rather than trying to hide from the truth that real mental balance can ever be truly achieved.

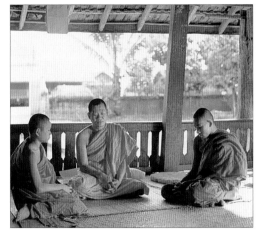

EASTERN MEDITATION
Part of the Eastern philosophy for mental good health involves reaching inner peace through meditation.

Eastern philosophies also emphasize the role of stability in providing the basis for a happy, contented life. They hold that we all share an innate balance of harmonious energy forces and that our task is to preserve this, avoiding excess in all things. This sense of balance is most famously illustrated in the concept of yin and yang, the two forces of energy thought to exist in all aspects of life. Taoists believe that these two forces are opposites, yin being passive, cold, and dark, and yang being active, warm, and light. Both forces are equally necessary, however, and reflect a mutual dependency. An excess of yang energy leads to aggression and destruction, while an excess of yin can cause inactivity. The balanced person aims for the middle path between extremes.

CHARACTERISTICS OF MENTAL WELL-BEING

All theories of good mental health propose that an individual must accept the realities of existence while still focusing on positive qualities. Finding a balance can be difficult; some signs of mental well-being include

▶ *Self-confidence and a sense of self-worth*

▶ *The ability to express emotions freely*

▶ *Overcoming of childish needs and wishes; the ability to tolerate frustration*

▶ *Independence of thought and action*

▶ *Ability to value and appreciate others*

▶ *Willingness to forgive others*

▶ *Living and thinking creatively*

▶ *Resolution of unconscious conflicts*

▶ *Ability to form and maintain close and intimate relationships*

▶ *Feeling comfortable in one's own company*

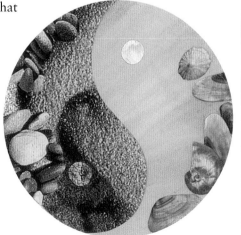

YIN AND YANG
The yin and yang symbol of balance reflects the sense of completeness that a person should ideally feel and express.

EMOTIONAL BEHAVIOR

Despite our best attempts to think rationally, strong emotions sometimes dominate our thinking. Researchers are looking at the extent to which it is possible to control powerful feelings.

States of arousal
Research has shown that different emotions have different physiological effects. Anger, for example, raises body temperature, whereas fear reduces it, and most emotions involve an increase in heart rate.

The field of emotions is a complex and controversial one, but researchers agree that humans do appear to share the same basic emotions of anger, happiness, sadness, and fear—regardless of culture or race. Studies have shown that people in different cultures will identify the same emotions when studying the facial expression of a person in a photograph. There is also evidence to suggest that facial expressions for basic emotions are actually inborn rather than acquired through experience or knowledge. In research conducted by the psychologist Carroll Izard in 1989, it was discovered that babies are capable of facially expressing pain, interest, and disgust from the moment of birth.

INSTINCTS AND EMOTIONS
Some researchers believe that because humans experience similar basic emotions, our feelings are of biological origin and derive from basic instincts. They argue that we are biologically programmed to seek out pleasurable experiences that bring happiness and to avoid unpleasant experiences

that produce fear or anger. According to this theory, experiencing the emotion of love might be motivated by your sex drive, while feeling jealousy might be motivated by your need for safety and security.

Lending further support to the argument that emotions are at least in part biologically determined is the fact that researchers have measured a number of different physiological reactions for different emotions. Anger, fear, and sadness, for example, can all produce a significant increase in heart rate, whereas depression can cause a slight decline in neural activity.

The relationship between physical response and emotional state makes sense in terms of our primitive survival instincts. Arousal of the nervous system prepares the body for "fight or flight" in a dangerous or threatening situation. If you are angry, you may decide to fight the source of the apparent threat, but if you are frightened, you may decide to run away. Either way, your nervous system will be aroused, increasing the flow of blood around your body, intensifying your levels of adrenaline, and tensing your muscles—all of which help your body to deal with the potential threat.

In contrast to anger and fear, some emotions can actually prevent arousal. Contentment, for example, can help to keep the body calm or reduce a state of agitation, and depression and boredom may slow down body processes even further. From this viewpoint it is easy to see how depression can become such a difficult cycle to break. As it lowers your state of arousal, it contributes to tiredness and general feelings of lethargy, making it even harder to motivate yourself and force a change in your perspective and outlook.

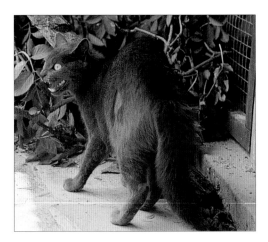

ANIMAL INSTINCTS
The way we physically respond to an emotion is an inherent part of our biological makeup. Like animals, we use facial expression, movement, and sounds to express our instinctive feelings.

WHAT IS BEHIND EMOTIONS?

Understanding the reasons behind your emotions may be one way you can come to a better understanding of destructive ones. For example, if your relationships are being adversely affected by possessiveness and jealousy, it may be useful to look at whether there is a more basic feeling of insecurity at work and what steps you can take to overcome this problem. Early experiences, such as rejection by or the death of a parent, may be causing insecurity, and confronting your past can help you to deal more effectively with the present.

THOUGHTS AND EMOTIONS

Despite the evidence for the importance of instinct in our emotions, there is also strong evidence that our moods may be influenced by our thoughts. By consciously deciding to behave in a happy way, the theory suggests, we can actually start to feel happy.

Research conducted by Fritz Stack in 1988 and subsequent experiments by Paul Ekman and Richard Davidson in 1993 have suggested that consciously willed behavior can alter your mood. Stack asked volunteers to hold a pen between their lips for a substantial amount of time. He found that, depending on whether the pen forced their mouths into a happy or sad expression, the volunteers actually started to feel happier or sadder. Holding a "happy" smile, produced by gripping a pen with the teeth, caused brain activity similar to that of a spontaneous smile at a pleasurable event; holding the muscles in a "sad" position increased feelings of depression.

Although simply forcing yourself to smile when you feel sad will not completely change your mood, it may help to regulate the emotional experience and possibly even inhibit it. This is a powerful argument for the effectiveness of positive thinking.

INDIVIDUAL DIFFERENCES

In addition to thoughts, other factors can profoundly influence your personal experience of emotion. Your own biological makeup will affect to an extent how intensely you feel emotions and how freely you express them. Scientific research suggests that we inherit particular patterns of temperament, emotions, and personality. A natural predisposition to an excessively active nervous system, for example, may increase the likelihood of a more emotional, highly strung personality, and a volatile and intensely emotional parent may produce a child with similar characteristics. However,

FACIAL EXPRESSIONS AND MOOD
Purposely adopting a certain facial expression can help to alter mood. By manipulating muscles in a particular way, you can simulate the associated feeling.

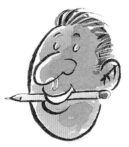

Gripping a pen between your teeth puts the muscles into a smiling expression and may help to improve mood.

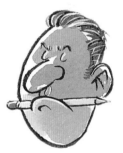

Holding a pen between your lips may lead to a feeling of sadness and depressed mood.

HOW LIE DETECTORS WORK

Polygraphs, or lie detectors, work by measuring emotional and bodily reactions. As a person answers a series of questions, the machine detects changes in heart rate, blood pressure, respiration, and perspiration. The theory behind the detector's effectiveness is that a person will react emotionally, and thus with increased physiological arousal, if he or she is not telling the truth.

The problem with this kind of test is that it does not allow for differences in psychological makeup. Some innocent people may become so nervous and physiologically aroused by the experience that they exhibit the same bodily responses as those anticipated of a guilty person. Conversely, some people, perhaps with the aid of drugs, are able to assert such control over their emotions that they can actually inhibit physical responses, thus tricking the machine. The results from lie detector tests can never be entirely conclusive, and other evidence is always needed in determining guilt or innocence.

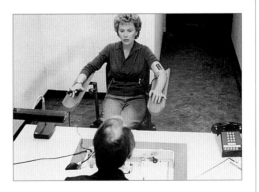

TESTING TIME
A baseline of physiological response is first established by asking neutral questions; the machine then detects deviations from this.

POPEYE AND OLIVE OYL
Stereotypes of gender difference can be found throughout popular culture. Characters like Popeye often reinforce social images, but opinions differ as to whether they actually construct them.

GENDER DIFFERENCE

For years people have argued over the apparently different makeup of men and women. While some people claim that there is an inherent physiological difference in the emotional responses of the sexes to certain situations, others claim that such ideas are a myth, brought about by sociocultural conditioning. Example: Boys allegedly are more aggressive, whereas girls are more sensitive and emotional. The truth of these different suppositions is very difficult to determine, and cultural, sociological, and historical factors all need to be taken into consideration. It is impossible, of course, to extricate the truth from all of these influences. If a girl is told from an early age that she has softer feelings than her brother and if she is exposed to media and advertising that confirm she must be soft, it will be very difficult for her not to conform to this stereotype.

Nevertheless, scientific research has shown that males do have greater quantities of hormones identified with aggression. The hormone testosterone, for example, which is more prevalent in the male body, is now known to affect the area of the brain that determines violent behavior. This fact may account for the common assumption that men are generally more violent than women or that they are more easily aroused to action and less passive. Such research cannot explain, however, individual dispositions toward certain characteristics or the variations in personality in both men and women.

Hypnosis
Many people testify to the power of hypnotism to subliminally influence a person's thoughts, so that even when returned to full consciousness, the body continues to feel and respond to what it was told under the state of hypnotic trance. Such therapy can arguably be useful in treating such addictions as smoking because it encourages people to believe in a newfound power, but many experts believe it is better to develop conscious self-control.

other factors such as upbringing are equally important in affecting how we behave and feel. If your parents were demonstrative and tended to express their emotions freely, for example, you are likely to do the same. Cultural background is also very important. In some cultures the public expression of emotion is discouraged. Differences in accepted behavior for men and women contribute yet another factor. Traditionally, in many cultures women have been allowed to be more open about their feelings, while men have been encouraged to suppress their feelings and to "act like a man."

Therapists agree that repressing emotions tends to be unhealthy because unresolved or unexpressed strong feelings may gain expression in other, more destructive forms. For example, tension headaches may be a sign of unexpressed anger or frustration. If you find it difficult to express feelings freely, therapy aimed at overcoming particular inhibitions—whether they are cultural, biological, or related to your particular experiences—may help.

Ways of managing your emotions

Emotions are very complex interactions of various factors, and although it is not always possible to control them—indeed, repressing them can be harmful in the long term—it is not always the best course to allow your emotions unbridled expression. Following are some strategies for helping you to manage emotions when you feel overwhelmed or out of control.

First, remember that how you behave can affect the intensity of what you feel. Extreme reactions, like slamming a door in anger, can actually make you feel angrier.

Second, keep in mind that you are physically aroused when you experience any strong emotions, so allow time for your physical response to calm down before taking any action. The old adage that you should slowly count to 10 when you're feeling angry is actually helpful.

Third, remember that your thoughts can influence your feelings, so try to be objective when assessing the situation that is upsetting you. (Chapters 6 and 7 explore in greater detail therapies for helping you to manage your emotions.)

INTROVERT OR EXTROVERT?
There can be little doubt that some people are naturally more outgoing or more retiring than others. Although social and cultural expectations may influence some of the characteristics that you have, there are many scientific theories that classify and determine certain people types. One of the most familiar studies was devised by the British psychologist Hans Eysenck. He

argued that a person's inherited biological makeup interacts with environmental factors, such as upbringing and schooling, to produce a basic personality type. Each type has a location on an emotional chart that contains a series of continuous dimensions.

The first dimension, known as the introversion-extroversion scale, reflects the degree to which a person directs energy toward himself or herself or to the outside world. For example, someone whose characteristics place him or her toward the end of the introversion scale is more reserved, while a person placed toward the extroversion end is more sociable and outgoing.

The second dimension concerns neuroticism and emotional stability. Essentially, it refers to an individual's tendency to become upset easily or to remain calm. The common traits of neuroticism include anxiety, depression, and guilt, whereas the behaviors associated with emotional stability include calmness and an even temper.

Eysenck believed that with a combination of the two dimensions people could be classified into one of four basic types. A shy, anxious person, for example, would be in

the introverted-neurotic section of the chart, while a quiet yet relatively calm person would be in the introverted-stable portion. Similarly, an outgoing but rather fearful person would be in the extroverted-neurotic section, and an easygoing extrovert would be labeled extroverted-stable.

Furthermore, in Eysenck's picture every individual has a number of characteristics and surface traits that can be found in his or her corresponding personality type (see chart below). For example, an impulsive, excitable person would be classified as extroverted-neurotic, while a thoughtful, passive, and generally reliable person would fall into the introverted-stable category.

Eysenck developed his theory in greater complexity, but his basic principles of personality type reveal remarkable similarities to those of ancient Greek theories. The famous doctor and philosopher Hippocrates proposed that characteristics are dictated by excesses of particular fluids, or "humors," of the body. These four fundamental qualities relate to the basic elements of all life but, as in Eysenck's theory, also identify common personality types and behaviors.

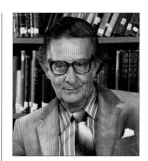

HANS EYSENCK (1916–1997)
Hans Eysenck developed the theory that both biological and cultural factors contribute to a basic personality type.

THE HUMORS

Hippocrates believed that excesses of any of the four fundamental elements of existence—earth, water, fire, and air—dictated personality types. Earth was said to be related to black bile and the melancholic disposition of a person. Water was identified with phlegm and reflected adaptability and listlessness. Fire related to the blood and sanguinity of a person, including happiness and optimism. Finally, air was associated with yellow bile and identified the choleric person who could be irritable and impulsive. Of course, such classifications don't allow for the complexity of individual variations, but it is interesting to note the correspondences between these categories and those devised by Eysenck.

PERSONALITY TYPES
Eysenck's theory of human personality (outer ring) shows remarkable overlap with the basic character types devised by the Greek physician Hippocrates (inner circle).

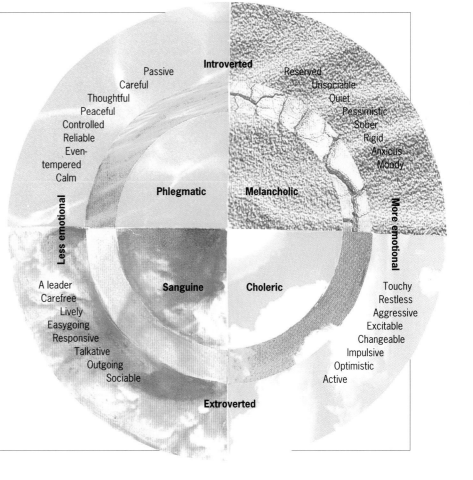

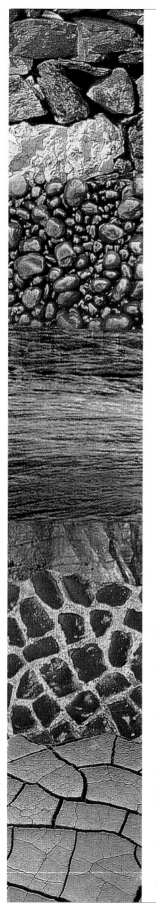

ASSESSING YOUR EMOTIONAL HEALTH

Consider the questions below and your natural responses to common situations. Everybody feels and behaves differently at different times, but think about how you would *normally* react to a situation.

Do not try to figure out what might be the correct answer but rather what is most indicative of you. Then check the information below the chart to see how emotionally healthy you are.

	QUESTIONS	SELDOM OR NEVER	SOMETIMES	OFTEN
1	Are you able to express your feelings easily?			
2	Do you feel reasonably happy most of the time?			
3	Do you have a sense of self-worth?			
4	Do you think people know the real you?			
5	Are you able to turn to someone when you feel upset?			
6	When angry with someone, can you tell that person?			
7	Do you generally feel able to stand up for yourself?			
8	Do you have a positive view of the future?			
9	Are you able to cope easily when things do not go your way?			
10	Do you feel relatively secure most of the time?			
11	Do you feel valued by your friends and family?			
12	Are you pleased with most of your achievements?			
13	Do you enjoy socializing with different people?			
14	Are you able to let yourself depend on someone?			
15	Do you have a good relationship with your family?			
16	As a child, were your feelings paid attention to?			
17	Do you find it easy to adapt to situations?			
18	Do you admire other people?			
19	Do you have ambitions and often set yourself goals?			
20	Are you able to accept change to your way of life?			
21	Do you try to avoid worrying about things?			
22	Do you feel that your life is essentially complete?			
23	Do you have a satisfying sexual relationship?			
24	Do you like your body?			

If you answered "often" to more than 10 of these questions, you probably have overall good emotional health. More answers in the "sometimes" column suggests that things need a little improvement and you should give some thought to why you are feeling negative. If you answered "seldom or never" more than 10 times, you need to assess your sense of control. Think about the causes of your discontent and ways in which you can improve your outlook.

UNDERSTANDING THE MIND

There are numerous ideas about what makes a person mentally, emotionally, and psychologically healthy, and many factors play a role in determining how each individual copes with life.

For centuries people have argued over the roles of biology and environment in determining character. Many have claimed that we are born with an innate personality that cannot be altered, while others have suggested that human character is more a product of experiences, and still others have proposed that a combination of these two influences character.

The biological theory suggests that the greatest influence on personality is what has been inherited, that genetics largely determine if a person will suffer psychological or emotional problems later in life. Manic depression and Schizophrenia, for example, are thought to be hereditary. We know that levels of certain chemicals and hormones in the brain can influence mood. People whose chemical makeup includes lower quantities of serotonin, one of the chemicals that transmit information in the nervous system, are more prone to depression, for instance. The biological view implies that they were born with lower levels.

Environmental theories focus on the role of experiences in shaping personality and attitudes. Having a healthy mind is said to be determined largely by external influences of childhood. A child who is repeatedly punished for laziness, for example, is more likely to feel guilt and inflict self-punishment in adulthood. Today opinion tends toward the view that both genetic and external aspects bear some influence.

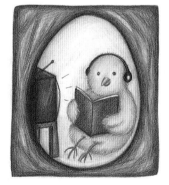

SEROTONIN
This polarized micrograph, magnified many times, shows molecules of serotonin, one of the brain's most important neurotransmitters. People who have adequate levels of serotonin are generally optimistic, creative, calm, and focused.

THREE THEORIES OF PERSONAL DEVELOPMENT

There are three basic theories about the influences that determine personality traits and character. Two of them focus primarily on one factor—either the genetic or the environmental. The third one, that a combination of these two forces is the basis for each person's behavior and emotions, is the most prevalent.

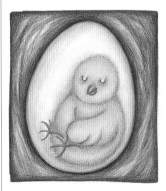

Biological theories propose that we genetically inherit most of our personal characteristics and our disposition.

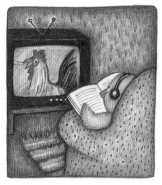

Environmental theories assert that we are conditioned largely by external forces and personal experiences as we develop.

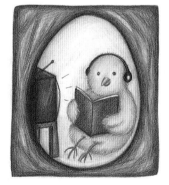

Combination theories are based on the premise that we are emotionally conditioned by both genetic and external influences.

WARTIME SEPARATION
Many children who were evacuated from danger zones—and separated from their families— during World War II suffered anxiety problems later in life. Some individuals had more difficulty in forming emotional attachments because the trauma of their early separation from parents was never confronted or resolved.

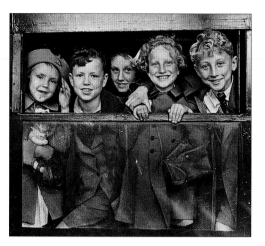

There is evidence for the combined view in the fact that many people who have had the same childhood experiences lead different adult lives. Of three children in a family with nurturing parents, two may lead successful lives and establish loving families of their own, while the third may develop deep psychological problems. The degree to which nature or nurture holds sway may never be fully resolved, but we are finding more ways to balance the two. Someone with a difficult childhood, for example, will not necessarily suffer emotional problems later in life if he or she receives therapy and guidance. Similarly, people who have learned to think negatively can learn to reprogram themselves once they recognize their habits of thinking. Even biochemical

disorders can be treated with drugs and therapy. It seems that a great many problems can be resolved with the right attention and therapeutic approach.

EVIDENCE FOR MENTAL HEALTH

Providing evidence for the various theories of what influences mental health is difficult. Only by having an understanding of what is mentally good can a therapist determine what is wrong, and studies are necessarily slow and long-term. A particular difficulty is that most scientific proof requires repetition of results, but every individual is different and so has a unique psyche and set of problems. Nevertheless, scientists have spent years doing research and documenting the results, attempting to provide concrete proof for their psychological theories.

The psychoanalyst John Bowlby made numerous studies of children who were evacuated from British cities during the Second World War. His evidence suggests that many of them suffered separation anxiety and had difficulty in forming personal attachments later in life. These conclusions could be drawn because the individuals were compared with others who had remained with their families and who were found to be generally more secure in adulthood.

Experiments have shown that if an animal is regularly subjected to a painful stimulus, it will learn to avoid the object or behavior

LITTLE PETER AND BEHAVIOR THERAPY

In the 1920s, John B. Watson conducted experiments in conditioning a child to be afraid of a rat. Following this research, Mary Cover-Jones developed ideas on curing children of their phobias. She devised a concept called behavioral therapy, which aimed to replace problematic behaviors with well-adjusted ones. Her

subject was a three-year-old boy named Peter who had an acute fear of furry objects. Cover-Jones set about curing his phobia by gradually bringing a rabbit near him during mealtimes. Through learning to associate the pleasure of food with the animal, Peter overcame his negative associations.

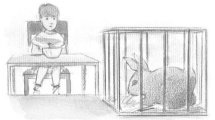

STAGE ONE
While Peter ate his favorite food, a caged rabbit was brought into distant view at the end of the room.

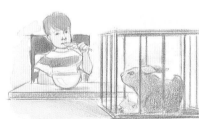

STAGE TWO
Every day the animal was inched a little closer while Peter ate his food and became accustomed to its presence.

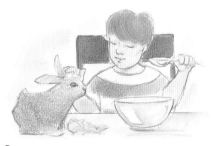

STAGE THREE
After two months Peter's tolerance had improved sufficiently to enable him to have the uncaged rabbit next to him.

that provokes the pain. Such research demonstrates how repeated exposure to something negative or painful can reinforce patterns of poor behavior. The evidence also suggests that set patterns of the mind can be adjusted. Many therapists believe that if it is possible to change the way you react, you can improve your emotional health as well by developing positive thoughts.

THEORIES AND THERAPIES

Of the hundreds of theories about mental and emotional health, a few have made exceptional contributions to the way we think about ourselves. Although superficially very different, these philosophies all have in common a belief that there is a direct correlation between the human psyche and the soul. Some suggest that it is only through truth and self-knowledge that a person can achieve inner balance and happiness.

Freudian theories

Embraced by some and scorned by others, Freudian psychoanalysis provides the basis for much of our modern understanding of the mind while remaining one of the most controversial areas of mental health. The concept developed by Sigmund Freud (1856–1939) is based on the significance of the unconscious psyche to overall mental health. Freud suggested that bad experiences or sensations are stored in the subconscious part of the mind and tend to inhibit personal development and fulfillment. He believed that bringing the subconscious thoughts, memories, and feelings into the open allows a person to work through anxieties and resolve deep conflicts. The role of the psychoanalyst is to help patients overcome their own mental resistance and confront and release the truth of their inner world.

While much of Freud's writing focuses on the unhealthy parts of the personality, his ultimate aim was to help people to understand themselves better and thus feel freer to choose the lives they wished to lead. He believed that avoiding the truth adds to a person's suffering and that only by facing deeply buried fears and feelings from the past can inner peace be achieved.

Through his extensive research into psychoanalysis, Freud sought to assist people in recognizing and addressing the anxieties and problems that they had concealed through repression. Chapter 6 looks at

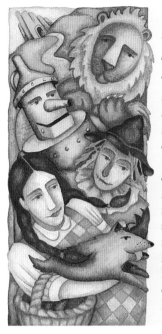

Fables and behavior

THE WIZARD OF OZ

The characters in the film *The Wizard of Oz* embody many of the classic qualities represented in Carl Jung's archetypes. The orphaned, innocent child Dorothy begins a journey that brings self-enlightenment and the conquest of good over evil. The Tin Man, Cowardly Lion, and Scarecrow, meanwhile, are all seeking qualities that symbolically represent universal human instincts and anxieties. The Tin Man's heart, the Scarecrow's brain, and the Lion's courage all reflect basic and essential human preoccupations with love, wisdom, and fortitude.

some of the theories and techniques that Freud devised in trying to help patients confront their repressed anxieties and emotions.

Jungian theories

Carl Jung (1875–1961), who studied with Freud, eventually rejected many of his teacher's theories, but he did believe in the role of the unconscious psyche and the importance of reconciling it with conscious thought. He proposed that there is a "collective unconscious" that is shared by all humanity and reflects a common development in evolutionary growth. Within this common psyche is a set of archetypes that represent shared human experiences and that express preoccupations and instincts. Such recognized figures as the innocent child, nurturing mother, and wise old man reveal how we look at the world outside ourselves and indicate our unconscious desire to identify with it. Well-known themes from mythology, such as the quest for the Holy Grail and Jason and the Golden Fleece, together with fairy tales, suggest that these archetypes are universal and can be found in cultures around the world.

Jung also described two archetypes, anima and animus, that represent the female and male qualities of each person. He believed that both characteristics reside within an individual and need to be acknowledged. By reconciling these opposites, a person can heal psychological divisions and achieve a greater sense of inner peace.

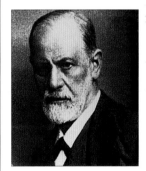

SIGMUND FREUD
The father of psychoanalysis, Freud developed many ideas that still influence psychology.

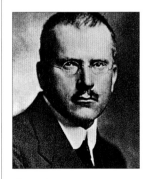

CARL JUNG
Initially a disciple of Freud, Jung went on to develop his own highly influential theories on the human mind.

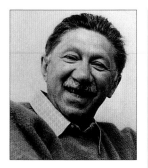

ABRAHAM MASLOW
*Conceptualizing the idea
of the peak experience,
Maslow claimed that it
is possible to reach a
stage of intense joy and
wonder.*

Unlike Freud, however, Jung believed that people naturally achieve a greater sense of unity and wholeness as they grow older. He saw middle and old age as a fruitful period in which past conflicts and unhappiness can be resolved. In contrast, Freud maintained that older people were unable to undo conflicts that had been formed in the early parts of their lives without psychoanalysis.

Maslow and self-actualization

One of the most successful attempts at establishing the link between emotional needs and personal development was developed in the 1950s and 1960s by the sociologist Abraham Maslow. His famous theory of self-actualization was devised principally in relation to people living in the developing world, but it can be equally well applied to people in the West. Maslow suggested that every person has a series of needs—ranging from basic requirements like food and shelter to psychological needs, such as achieving your full potential. For those at the bottom level, the pursuit of basic needs is the over-riding concern, leaving little time to satisfy other desires. Once people are able to establish a degree of self-sufficiency so that their basic needs are met, they can focus their attention on satisfying their emotional desires, such as building intimate friendships and self-esteem and accomplishing things.

Everyone's ultimate goal, according to Maslow, is to achieve the top stage of self-actualization and enjoy the benefits of a rich emotional life, with a good perception of reality and a healthy acceptance of people—known as a peak experience.

Bach flower remedies

Edward Bach was a doctor and homeopath who believed that there is a strong relationship between a patient's illnesses and state of mind. He argued that the true cause of physical sickness lay within the negative attitudes that people have toward both themselves and life in general. Bach claimed that through the various circumstances and experiences of our lives, we tend to lose sight of our direction and acquire negative

MASLOW'S PYRAMID

According to Abraham Maslow, our individual and collective needs are all part of a hierarchy. Only when we have satisfied our basic requirements—such as obtaining food and shelter and feeling secure and loved—can we then fulfill our higher aspirations. Self-actualization occurs when all the fundamental motivations of existence have been attained and we go on to realize our creative potential.

HIERARCHY OF NEEDS
Feeling safe, loved, and fulfilled will enable us to move on to an even higher sense of completeness.

Self-actualization, achieving one's full potential, including creative activities

Self-esteem needs, involving prestige and feelings of accomplishment

Belonging and love needs, such as intimate relationships and friendships

Security needs, including safety

Physiological needs, such as food, warmth, water, and rest

Self-fulfillment needs

Psychological needs

Basic needs

emotional symptoms, such as depression and irritability. He proposed that contentment is possible only by developing those characteristics that make us truly aware of our individuality and that restore a sense of balance.

Bach developed a series of 38 flower remedies for treating the negative attitudes behind a whole range of emotional and physical disorders. He believed that his plant remedies contained natural "vibrations" that help to restore mental harmony.

At the heart of Bach therapy is the need for an individual to identify the emotion or mental state that is causing the problem. For example, one remedy, mimulus, is recommended for anxiety, but if the underlying cause of the anxiety is actually irritation or anger, a different remedy will be recommended. Essentially, Bach believed that each person needs to think through his or her emotions and motivations and be open and honest in self-assessment. (Pages 74–75 provide more information on Bach's theories, including many of his remedies.)

Polarity therapy

Polarity therapy was devised at the beginning of the 20th century by Dr. Randolph Stone. It embraces the Eastern concept of yin and yang and emphasizes the balance between mind and body. According to Dr. Stone's theory, we are all made up of energy that flows cyclically from positive to negative sources. This energy needs to flow freely in order to link physical, emotional, psychological, and spiritual levels. Pain and illness—whether physical or emotional—are caused by blockages in this dynamic.

According to polarity theory, different areas of the body relate to the various elements of existence: ether governs the voice, hearing, and throat; water is the generative force that dictates emotion; air relates to the lungs; fire relates to the digestive system; and earth is identified with the rectum and bladder. Energies need to flow freely among these components, and polarity therapists encourage free current by setting up negative and positive poles with their hands. With the help of massage, manipulation, diet, and exercise, clients should achieve a greater sense of balance and efficient functioning.

Dr. Stone also strongly believed in the link between mind and body, claiming that "as we think, so we are." In other words, if we think negative thoughts about

IT'S GOOD TO TALK

Talking and being open with others can enhance both emotional and physical health. In one study at the University of Miami, a group of students was asked to recall and talk about stressful or traumatic experiences that had affected their lives. The events chosen were to be ones brought into the open for the first time and not discussed previously with anybody else. It was found that those students who were the most honest in their revelations enjoyed better health for the following six months, whereas students who were reserved in what they revealed were subsequently more prone to a weak immune system and general ill health. Although such evidence can never be entirely conclusive, it does suggest that expressing your feelings will help you at least to relax physically and emotionally and will result in a greater sense of control and direction in your life.

ourselves, we are more likely to suffer physical and emotional disorders. Part of the therapy devised by Stone aims to improve self-awareness and emotional understanding. As in many Eastern philosophies, the essential belief is that when balance is achieved in both physical and mental activity, the entire body and mind will be able to attain a state of harmonious equilibrium.

Buddhism

Although there are several different branches of Buddhism, the basic principle of striving for enlightenment is the same in all of them. The practice of ethics and meditation is said to lead eventually to a state of psychological happiness and to insight and understanding of the nature of existence.

It is thought that the original Buddha, Siddhartha Gautama, was born in about 563 B.C., although in Buddhist belief he had already passed countless previous lives in spiritual practice. After living a relatively secular lifestyle, which included a wife and

POLARITY THERAPY
Polarity therapy aims to improve energy flow throughout the body. In the "tummy rock," the practitioner's hands provide a positive and negative charge between the head and stomach as he or she gently rocks the patient's torso.

THE BUDDHA
The name Buddha *means "Enlightened One" and denotes the ability to reach a transcendental state of wisdom, compassion, energy, and happiness.*

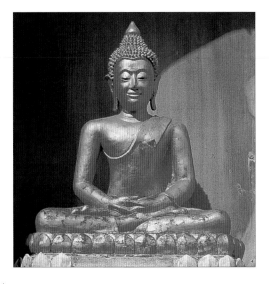

son, Siddhartha went off to pursue a nomadic life of austerity and reflection. While sitting under a fig tree, he attained full insight into the nature of the world and became the Buddha—the Enlightened One.

The Buddha then taught others how to gain enlightenment. Claiming to be restoring rather than developing a faith, Buddha disseminated the insight that all existence is impermanent. He demonstrated that humanity is free to reshape destiny and that by taking the "Middle Path" in life—practicing generosity, ethical behavior, meditation, and reflection—an individual can attain a state of illuminated consciousness. According to Buddhist belief, this is the ultimate happiness and goal of human life. (See pages 143–148 for more information on Buddhism.)

HELPING YOURSELF
Most people today accept that experiences from their past in some way influence their present and future. Just as some mental illnesses are related to early experiences, so a happy, content adulthood is often associated with security in childhood. But the totality of childhood need not prescribe how a person copes with adulthood. Taking responsibility for your feelings and accepting that the past is affecting you can help you come to terms with your experiences. Similarly, using the mind to improve emotional and physical well-being is also important.

Taking steps to make yourself fit, happy, and confident will enable your mind and body to work in harmony. People who are generally anxious or who have low self-esteem tend to be more vulnerable to tension, which in turn can accentuate their helplessness. Simply believing in yourself can help you to enjoy a healthier, happier life.

THE POWER OF MIND OVER ILLNESS

There have been many documented medical cases in which patients with serious, even life-threatening illnesses have apparently willed themselves to better health. One example is that of the American holistic therapist Louise Hay, author of the book, *You Can Heal Your Life.* Accepting her disease as a life-changing experience, she fought her own cancer using affirmations, visualization, nutritional cleansing, and psychotherapy to cleanse herself both mentally and physically. Hay developed a positive frame of mind in which she felt able to "think herself well." She now teaches, writes, and lectures all over the world about her experiences and her philosophy for maintaining good health with positive thinking.

Although every person's attitude and health status varies, believing in one's own ability to relax and be healthy will obviously be beneficial. Simply feeling that you have some control can make an enormous difference. Although you should always seek professional help for serious illness, trying to assist the healing process yourself can be very beneficial.

A technique that many people find helpful is to imagine their immune system at work. Visualizing an efficient system fighting off illness can strengthen your belief in the body's fitness and its natural ability to heal itself. Picturing the white blood cells attacking foreign invaders, for example, and defeating germs that can potentially cause harm provides a sense of empowerment. This confidence in turn provides a sense of calmness and makes you feel less prone to the debilitating physical effects of stress. By improving your mental and emotional outlook, you can enhance your physical health.

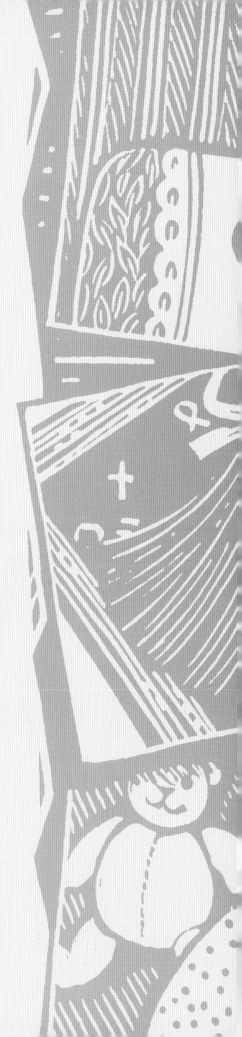

CHAPTER 2

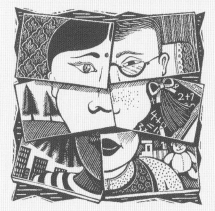

HEALTHY EMOTIONAL DEVELOPMENT

The way in which we develop as individuals affects the way we cope with daily life. As we accumulate experiences and as our expectations are met or not, we learn to adjust our outlook and behavior. This chapter looks at emotional development and some of the pressures that commonly affect us in different stages of life.

EMOTIONS AND THE CHILD

The experiences of childhood play a significant role in forming adult character. How children learn to deal with events and their feelings will affect the way they mature emotionally.

Natural expression
The emotions of happiness, anger, and sadness are with us from the moment of birth.

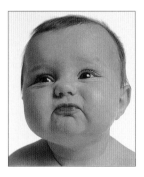

GRIMACE OF NECESSITY
Babies naturally express pain and distress in order to convey their survival needs.

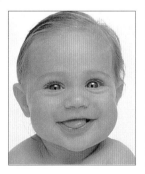

SMILE OF JOY
Pleasure is an innate sensation that results from our contentment when basic needs have been fulfilled.

As adults, we use the word *emotion* to describe such feelings as anger, sadness, happiness, discontent, and fear, and we often express them with words. Babies cannot communicate their feelings through language, but they are still capable of feeling a whole range of emotions and of expressing them by crying, grimacing, or smiling. In fact, many scientists believe that most of the emotions experienced and expressed by a baby are innate qualities that are present at birth. Crying because of discomfort comes naturally and is a fairly common response to the sudden change of environment experienced in the first few moments after birth.

However, babies are born with a limited range of emotions compared to those felt by a normal, healthy adult. While such feelings as pride or guilt have no place in a newborn's life, a baby does need the primitive sensations of fear, happiness, and displeasure, all of which help to ensure survival. An infant's first sensations are largely linked to hunger, tiredness, and discomfort. The point at which a child's impulses become what we would conventionally describe as emotions is difficult to determine. Acknowledging his or her mother as a separate entity suggests that a baby is truly an emotional being who is capable of experiencing feelings of attachment, separation, and loss.

In addition to innate emotions, babies are born with the need to form certain attachments in order to thrive both physically and psychologically. Insecure attachment can occur for a number of reasons. A lack of continuity in the people who care for a baby, for example, may result in an inhibited child who is frightened to explore the surrounding environment or a child who is unruly and difficult. If such inhibitions and

TAOISM AND HUMAN POTENTIAL

Taoist doctrine teaches that we are all born possessing the "Three Treasures" (*san bao*) of life: essence, energy, and spirit (*jing, chi, and shen*), which exist in perfect balance with one another. Our prenatal heritage is an innate potential to lead a satisfying life. After birth the three elements become subject to the temporal, human world and can be put out of balance. When loss of equilibrium occurs, it causes emotional poverty and physical ill health. By striving to restore harmony among the Three Treasures, however, we may still realize our potential.

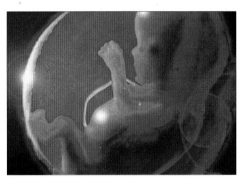

THE PERFECT BEING
Taoists believe that before birth we exist in harmony with the universe. The key to our happiness lies in restoring this balance.

DID YOU KNOW?
A baby's earliest smiles are made with the use of a single muscle. As the interaction between mother and baby increases, however, the infant's emotions and physical responses become more complex.

behavior stay with an individual, they could develop into more complex problems and possible underachievement as an adult.

The issue of attachment is a complicated one. The ability to completely trust and depend on another human being is very important to mental well-being, and psychologists agree that babies need stable and reliable relationships to thrive. However, overly protective parenting can also be harmful and may prevent a child from developing strong self-esteem and confidence. Successful parenting relies on a delicate process of nurturing and providing love and support while gradually allowing a child to become self-reliant.

DEVELOPMENT FROM INFANCY TO ADULTHOOD

The rate at which a child grows physically and mentally is unsurpassed at any other time in life. The intensity of development varies during the first 18 years, but the experiences and emotions accumulate to form an astounding cognitive achievement.

From the earliest days of infancy, during which a baby recognizes only its own basic needs, a child grows to understand his or her independent self and acquires a comprehension of the surrounding world. Such development also involves feeling and recognizing most of the emotions that we are familiar with as adults. A baby's first encounter with separation, which might occur during weaning, for example, sets up a blueprint for the future experiences of attachment and loss. Similarly, the initial years, when toddlers learn that there are limits to what they are allowed to do, provide a foundation for the disappointments and irritations of later life. Even acknowledging and dealing with the presence of siblings introduces those first comprehensions of jealousy and love and the necessity of sharing.

As a child reaches adolescence and experiences the initial challenges of romantic love and divided loyalty, he or she will become more emotionally self-aware and complete but will still continue to grow. People never really stop changing, but most of their emotional development takes place during the first 18 years. It is for this reason that a child needs to be taken care of in a way that will support physical and mental health.

Individuals who fail to develop or are too rigidly protected from the realities of life may suffer from unnecessary anxiety or unresolved conflict. If a child is always discouraged from asserting individuality or from developing an identity separate from that of the parents, as an adult he or she may continue to fear the possibility of sudden rejection or independence. Most psychotherapists believe that the route to a mentally healthy adulthood lies in both experiencing and resolving the various emotional conflicts encountered during childhood.

The meaning of emotional maturity

Although normal people have developed an awareness of their emotions by adulthood, such consciousness is not necessarily synonymous with maturity. Many adults never achieve full emotional maturity and may even regress—particularly during moments of frustration—to infantile yearnings and behavior. Turning to food or drink in a

THE EFFECTS OF DAY CARE ON ATTACHMENT

Research differs as to the effects of day care on infant attachment and development. While the psychologist Jay Belsky suggests that it can be damaging to a child under the age of one, other analysts, like Bengt-Erik Andersson, claim that infants actually do better—developing social and cognitive skills much sooner.

Although such a debate may never be conclusively resolved, the quality of child care is obviously a key factor in developing attachment and a good emotional basis for later life. Caring attention and support are crucial to infant security, and finding a center that is well staffed, funded, and managed requires thorough research, keen observation, and sometimes a little bit of luck.

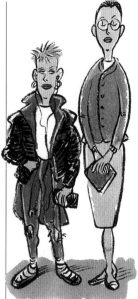

BIRTH ORDER
Some theorists believe that position in the family's birth order can affect personality. First-born children tend to be more reserved and conservative, forming close allegiances with their parents for fear of becoming displaced by younger siblings. Younger brothers or sisters are often observed to be more rebellious and outgoing, counteracting the oldest sibling's close adherence to the parents' expectations by being as different as possible.

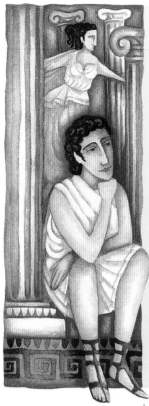

Fables and myths

OEDIPUS

Freud famously claimed that one of the first emotional conflicts experienced by a child occurs during sexual development. He said that as children become aware of their sexuality, they develop a specific attraction to the parent of the opposite sex. These emotions can lead to extreme protectiveness of that parent—such as a daughter not wishing to leave her father's side—or jealousy of the other parent. This so called Oedipus Complex is named after the hero of Greek mythology who was reputedly abandoned at birth. Not knowing the identity of his parents, Oedipus unwittingly killed his father and married his mother, thus fulfilling his latent sexual desires.

moment of pain, for example, echoes the way a distressed baby resorts to the breast or bottle for some oral comfort.

But emotional maturity is itself difficult to define. Having the mental ability to experience, acknowledge, and confront an entire range of emotions suggests that a person has good mental stability, but every individual must occasionally encounter new and over-

whelming situations. It is perhaps being able to meet and adequately deal with these new sensations that reflects emotional honesty.

Abandoning the childlike idea that things should be black or white and realizing that life need not work in exclusive opposites is a mark that a person has reached a greater understanding of self and society. A number of psychotherapists suggest that it is only when we realize the full complexity of our behavior and motivation that emotional maturity can be achieved.

Relating to others

From the moment that a newborn becomes aware of his or her own individuality, the pattern of relationships is set. The infant learns to recognize the separateness of other people and realize that mother will come and go and provide love and nourishment but also have her own existence.

Sharing the attention of an adult also introduces a child to the closeness as well as the competition that exists in all relationships. Accepting that a mother has other interests, for example, or that a younger sibling alters the focus of attention, provides mental preparation for the vast array of relationships, emotions, and experiences ahead. Learning to tolerate feelings of jealousy and frustration, as well as developing a sense of responsibility and concern for others, sets up an individual for the encounters and conflicts of adult life.

PIAGET'S STAGES OF COGNITIVE DEVELOPMENT

In the late 1920s Swiss psychologist Jean Piaget proposed the idea that children actually think in a different way than adults do. Although many specialists now reject some aspects of his theory, his basic principle of four key stages of development is still used as a guide for research.

The first stage lasts from birth to age 2 and is the time when infants learn about the relationship between themselves and others. The second stage, from age 2 to 7, is the period in which a child begins to form mental images. The third stage, from 7 to 11, involves learning to think in relational terms and comprehending size, relationships, and dimensions. The final stage, from 11 on, represents the beginning of both logical and abstract thought, enabling an individual to use intelligent and lateral thinking in adult life.

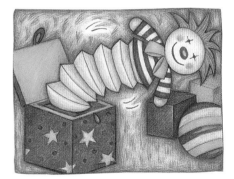

SENSORIMOTOR STAGE
Between birth and age 2, infants begin to learn the relationship between cause and effect. By manipulating objects, children learn that they can bring about specific reactions.

Most brothers and sisters go through periods of closeness and quarreling as they grow up, experiencing the emotions of their maturing individuality and the realities of sharing parental attention and the family home. These conflicts rarely have a lasting effect on the siblings' long-term relationship, although they can be very trying for parents at the time.

Things should never be allowed to get out of hand, but most experts agree that interference generally makes things worse and many arguments are actually best left to the children to resolve. Nevertheless, expressing your disapproval of the situation, without taking sides, can at least help siblings to realize that their actions are affecting the entire family. Suggesting strategies for resolving the problem is a good way to set up a framework for reconciliation. Rather than having a solution imposed on them, children need to learn how to deal with sibling rivalry and to see arguments from different perspectives.

Ultimately, a supportive family unit is the best way to nurture and help a child understand the importance of relationships. By providing a broad range of experiences but also the supportive structure to deal with emotional development, a family can establish the foundation for a person to grow into a well-balanced adult. While a loving family is no guarantee of adult happiness, it does provide the best basis possible.

Stress and the child

As the major source of a child's mental good health, the family unit needs to be as stable as possible. Major upheavals within the home can expose children to a series of traumatic emotions, and a lack of support in these moments can lead to the threat of emotional imbalance later in life. How the family deals with the loss of a parent or another child, for example, can determine how well a child will develop emotionally. A supportive, comforting, open family is far more likely to help a youngster become well adjusted than one that does not provide the right circumstances for recovery.

Children's sense of security is based to a large extent on the integrity of the family unit; they feel personally threatened if the unit seems to be in danger. Arguing parents can be frightening and disruptive, implying that the home is in danger of breaking up and that the mother and father no longer love each other. In families in which parents were actually separating, many children have reported feeling lost or disoriented, as if their world were being destroyed.

While divorce is undeniably traumatic for everybody involved, children can and do recover from the breakup of the family home. A constantly tense, unhappy household can actually be more psychologically damaging and stressful than a family unit that is carefully split up to ensure that

continued on page 38

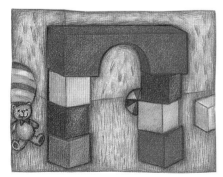

PREOPERATIONAL STAGE
From about age 2 to 7, children begin to form mental images and engage in make-believe play. They may, however, find it difficult to see the world from perspectives other than their own.

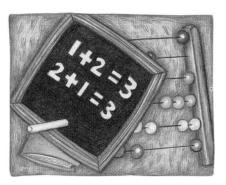

CONCRETE OPERATIONS
Between the ages of 7 and 11, the young mind starts to work more like an adult's as it begins to think in relational terms and understand the concept of reversing certain actions and behavior.

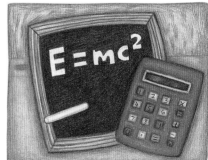

FORMAL OPERATIONS
From about age 11 on, children can think both abstractly and with logic, formulating general theories and hypotheses. These skills continue to develop throughout life.

Child Psychotherapist

If a child or adolescent is suffering from emotional or psychological disturbances, a child psychotherapist can assist the young person in dealing with the problems. Therapists help individuals come to terms with their thoughts and emotions.

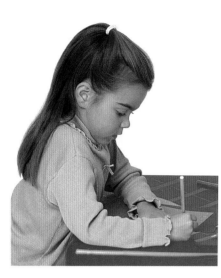

EMOTIONAL EXPRESSION
Therapy often involves encouraging a child to pursue a creative activity. Drawing is an excellent way to get a youngster to express emotions that are too difficult to articulate with language.

Child psychotherapists use different techniques according to the age and cognitive ability of their patients. Small children, who do not have access to sophisticated words or language, will be encouraged to play and express their anxieties in a behavior that is familiar to them. The therapist will sit with the child while he or she draws pictures, models clay, or selects toys and games. By observing what the child chooses and creates, how the child behaves and how focused and absorbed he or she is, the therapist can begin to understand the mental processes at work. Talking to the child about the game or artwork or toy also helps to draw out the child's inner reality. This can aid in identifying the significance of a particular plaything.

Therapy for teenagers is usually conducted in a series of brief sessions. The volatile, changing nature of adolescence normally requires several consultations to resolve a crisis quickly. Therapy is concerned with helping the young person to reflect on his or her inner and outer worlds in the safety of a private discussion with confidentiality guaranteed. Many teenagers feel under intense social pressure and scrutiny, and developing a space for private reflection where thought and expression will not be judged or criticized is very important. Anxieties

Origins

Anna Freud, the youngest daughter of the famous psychoanalyst Sigmund Freud, became his chief disciple. In the 1930s and 1940s she started using her father's theories of psychoanalysis with children. Although she established the fact that psychological problems can indeed affect the young, her application of adult techniques was often too sophisticated for her younger patients.

The psychoanalyst Melanie Klein, who was working around the same time as Anna Freud, developed the idea of play therapy. This proved helpful in accessing the deeper levels of a child's mind, and it forms the basis of much of today's therapy.

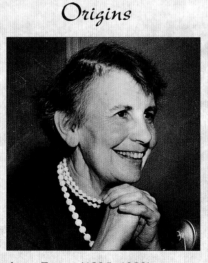

ANNA FREUD (1895–1982)
Anna Freud was one of the first people to recognize that children also have psychological problems.

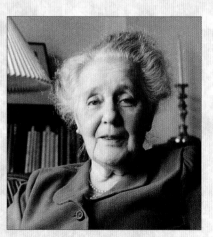

MELANIE KLEIN (1882–1960)
Melanie Klein developed play therapies specially designed to encourage the expression of emotion.

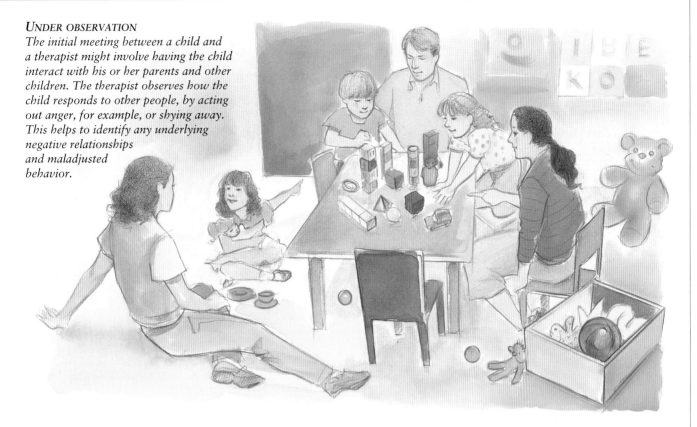

UNDER OBSERVATION
The initial meeting between a child and a therapist might involve having the child interact with his or her parents and other children. The therapist observes how the child responds to other people, by acting out anger, for example, or shying away. This helps to identify any underlying negative relationships and maladjusted behavior.

regarding sex, family relationships, or the future can make an adolescent very vulnerable, and the confidence of and close relationship with a therapist can make a big difference.

What training does a child psychotherapist have?

Child psychotherapists usually have at least a Ph.D. in child psychology, whereas child psychoanalysts have a medical degree and several years of postdoctoral study. This preparation usually includes infant and toddler observation, clinical and theoretical training, and personal analysis. It is very intensive and reflects the huge responsibility of providing psychological support.

How does child therapy fit into the caring profession?

Child therapists often work as part of a wider group of professionals who are concerned with the family and the protection and welfare of children and adolescents. Children and families may be referred to therapists through their doctors, social services, or teachers. Once

therapy has been decided on, all of these professionals work together to ensure that both the child and family get the appropriate help. They will also try to see that the child returns to normal life as soon as possible.

What kind of problems can be helped?

Small children can suffer from a wide range of problems, which are often expressed through nightmares, tantrums, bed-wetting, and phobias. Many of these behaviors are symptoms of a deeper anxiety that the therapist will try to identify and help the child to resolve.

Teenage problems usually involve depression or rebellious behavior, such as drug abuse, bullying, truancy, or pregnancy. Many high school and university students experience intense pressure during examinations, and therapy can help them to cope with spiraling stress.

Are the parents involved?

Although parents or other relatives may be involved in an initial consultation, they are not usually present

during therapy. Some problems, however, are linked to or shared by the whole family and must be addressed with all of the concerned members present. In such cases the therapist will often work with the family unit as a whole.

WHAT YOU CAN DO AT HOME

Parents can encourage their children to be more open about their feelings and anxieties by allowing them to express themselves without pressure or judgment. This may mean sitting alone with a child, away from family activities, and letting him or her talk freely or ask questions. Allowing a young child to play with toys or draw while you talk may help the youngster be more open and expressive.

If a child's behavior is worrying you or you feel that you cannot cope, do not be afraid to contact a therapist or guidance center. Accepting help does not mean failure; it is evidence that you acknowledge the existence of a problem and wish to do the best for your child.

HELPING A CHILD TO COPE WITH DIVORCE

Although family divorce will affect how and where a child or teenager lives, he or she usually has no control over these changes. Not surprisingly, many children become distressed at such disruption, and adolescents may feel confused or express intense anger. It is important to remember that you are not the only one feeling anger and distress; children also experience fear and, quite often, a sense of blame. Observing parents who are upset or angry can cause children to feel unwanted and possibly lead to disruptive or attention-seeking behavior. Openly discussing the implications of divorce, rather than enshrouding it in guilt and mystery, will help a child come to terms with the emotional upheaval more easily. The following ideas may help.

▶ *Avoid quarreling in the presence of your children or laying blame on each other.*

▶ *Try to stay calm and keep routines as normal as possible.*

▶ *Hide only the excesses of your feelings. Children need to know that they are not the only ones who are being affected emotionally. They also have to understand that they are not to blame for the breakup.*

▶ *Try to be generous with custody arrangements. Although doing so may be difficult, your children need to see you show respect for and encourage a smooth continuation of their relationship with your former spouse.*

MICHELANGELO'S DAVID
Commonly accepted as the prime example of manhood, the famous statue David *actually depicts the proportions of an adolescent. The figure's head, hands, and feet are slightly larger in proportion to his limbs and trunk than an adult's would be.*

nobody suffers further pain. While many parents feel that they need to stay together for the sake of the children, research indicates that divorce does not have to cause permanent emotional damage. If custody is handled amicably and children are kept suitably informed, most go on to live normal lives and have successful relationships. Furthermore, evidence suggests that the younger a child is at the time of a breakup, the sooner he or she is likely to recover. While preschool children, for example, may show signs of distress for about a year, teenagers can be affected for much longer.

THE CHALLENGES OF ADOLESCENCE

The transition from childhood to adulthood can be both exciting and terrifying. It is a crucial turning point for the individual, and emotional and physical development can cause confusion and insecurity during this period. The risk of psychological problems increases during adolescence; a serious illness like schizophrenia may emerge at this time.

Learning to cope with the physical changes of puberty can be one of the most difficult challenges. As breasts and genitalia develop, as pubic hair grows and menstruation begins, teenagers find themselves confronted with an unfamiliar body and a whole range of new insecurities. Although most girls begin to experience changes by about the age of 13 and boys by 15, earlier or later development is fairly common and can be a source of great anxiety and self-consciousness. The often deep-rooted desire of teenagers to fit in with their peers may be undermined by the sudden, very apparent differences among friends.

Furthermore, many teenagers are emotionally and intellectually unprepared for the large number of changes their bodies undergo. Fascination, embarrassment, even alarm can be common reactions as individuals increasingly develop sexual awareness.

As children begin to look more like adults, they also start to feel like them as well. Learning to deal with sexual attraction and the new kind of relationships that this brings can be very difficult. While reevaluating their friendships and shifting focus away from their parents, teenagers often feel increasingly insecure and lacking in confidence. The intensity of their feelings of love, anger, sadness, and elation can be disorienting too, and many young adolescents feel unable to piece together their various roles to form a coherent self.

The future is frighteningly unknown, and the reality of entering another stage of life with new responsibilities and self-awareness is daunting. Unsurprisingly, adolescence can be a time of immense emotional stress, and a supportive family unit can be of the utmost importance in helping an individual through the psychological minefield. Simply

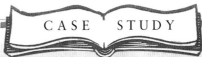
A Difficult Adolescent

Adolescence can be a time of great upheaval for both the individual and the entire family. How well this difficult period is negotiated will depend on the parents' relationship with their child and their own ability to cope with change. Teenagers often want increasing independence but they also still need to feel part of a secure and loving family unit.

Lisa is 16 and facing final examinations at school. She has always been a good student and is expected to do well, but her parents have noticed a sudden, disturbing change in her behavior; they are worried that she is jeopardizing her academic success. Lisa has been staying out late at night and has been warned about smoking on the school premises.

Lisa sits in stony silence at mealtimes and hardly touches her food. Her parents are increasingly concerned about the weight she has been losing but get only an angry response when they try to discuss it. Although Lisa admits she would like to relate to her parents as she used to, she often feels upset with them and insists that she just wants to be left alone.

WHAT SHOULD LISA'S PARENTS DO?

Rather than dwelling on the disappearance of Lisa's pleasant side, her parents need to remember that beneath the anger and rebellion there is still a vulnerable child. It is important to let an adolescent know that, despite all the arguments, you are still there to provide love and support and encouragement.

Teenagers do need boundaries, even though they may rebel against them, and the security and consistency of them can actually be comforting. Explaining why you have set rules and why keeping up with her studies will give her greater options for the future may help reduce some of Lisa's resentment and improve family relationships.

Action Plan

EATING HABITS
Use mealtimes as an opportunity to sit down and talk. Allow Lisa to prepare her own food occasionally to encourage her sense of being in control.

LIFESTYLE
Set boundaries that are strict but fair, such as allowing late nights on the weekends if weekdays have been spent keeping up with academic work.

EMOTIONAL HEALTH
Discuss problems as rationally as possible; establish an atmosphere of mutual respect and honesty.

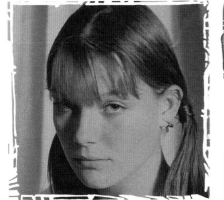

EATING HABITS
Teenagers can become fixated on their bodies and harm themselves. Extreme self-consciousness can lead to dangerous behavior.

LIFESTYLE
Pressures about doing well in school can cause some teenagers to rebel against studying altogether.

EMOTIONAL HEALTH
Pent-up frustration is often expressed in confrontation. Mixed feelings can be confusing.

HOW THINGS TURNED OUT FOR LISA

Although the situation did not change radically right away, Lisa did start to calm down. She agreed to participate in meals by preparing food that she wanted and sometimes choosing the topic of conversation at mealtimes. Gradually, the more relaxed atmosphere enabled her to talk more openly about her feelings of anger and insecurity. She also agreed to study harder during the week if she could keep her social life on the weekends.

NATURE OR NURTURE?

There is now evidence to suggest that a lot of teenage delinquency may actually have a biological basis. For example, adolescent boys who are prone to severe fits of temper and high levels of disobedience often have a particularly large amount of the hormone androstendione (a precursor to testosterone) in their blood. Teenage girls who have a relatively large amount of this hormone (although not as much as boys) can be more prone to defiant and angry behavior. Nevertheless, sociocultural influences also have an impact on how a teenager behaves.

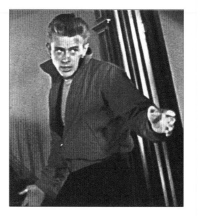

REBEL WITH A CAUSE?
James Dean portrayed the archetypal rebellious adolescent—the angst-ridden teenager who felt misunderstood and confused by the conflicting emotions of youth.

Common teenage problems

Given that teenagers are essentially young adults, the range of mental and emotional problems that can affect them is vast. Nevertheless, many recurring problems, such as the stress of studies, body self-consciousness, and depression are symptomatic of the period of transition that individuals must face at this age. Just as increasing sexuality brings anxiety, so growing awareness of the body can lead to obsessions with appearance and image. While adolescence is typically the age at which most people become aware of their looks, consciousness of the body can become obsessive and lead to eating disorders. (See page 118 for more detail on how to deal with these problems.)

At the same time that adolescents are experiencing drastic emotional and physical developments, they must also endure the pressures of getting good grades in school and making initial career decisions. How individuals respond to such pressures varies. While some young people seem to take everything in stride, others become intensely anxious or possibly even revolt against the expectations being placed upon them. A supportive, encouraging network of family and friends can do much to relieve some of the pressure. Teenagers need to know that they are loved and supported throughout these stressful times and that they do not have unrealistic expectations to live up to.

AROMATHERAPY
Teenage problems occasionally require professional help, but many stressful experiences can be relieved by simply promoting relaxation. Aromatic candles, for example, or relaxing music can help to instill calm.

looking back on your own adolescent experiences might help you remember what a difficult time it can be.

Teenage sexuality

As sexual awareness develops, it is common for teenagers to form crushes on teachers, pop stars, or even their parents' friends. Admiration can develop into more intense feelings of passion, reflecting the increasing maturity of the adolescent.

Many parents express concern over their teenagers' growing independence and find sex one of the most difficult problems to discuss openly. Enshrouding sex in mystery or placing unrealistic expectations on your child, however, can cause inhibition and discomfort later on. Being realistic about sexuality means setting boundaries but also accepting that your teenager is developing into a sexually mature adult.

Openly discussing the dangers and pitfalls, as well as the pleasures, of sex and the individual's own personal concerns can help to make the subject more understandable. Most parents would agree that it is better to have an honest relationship with their teenage son or daughter and know what is going on than to suffer embarrassment and encourage deceit. Many teenagers simply want answers, and being as open as possible will enable you to provide guidance.

PEER PRESSURE

Parents worry about the influences that peers can have on their teenage sons or daughters. In fact, though adolescence is the age during which people are most vulnerable to peer pressure, close friendships and groups do not necessarily lead to trouble and bad behavior. Most teenagers find that they are better at sharing their new experiences and feelings with friends of their own age, and the support that this sharing provides can be invaluable. Also, many adolescents encourage each other to achieve good grades or participate in activities that develop skills, and they provide constructive solutions to many common sources of adolescent anxiety and angst.

THE DEMANDS OF ADULTHOOD

Emerging from the turmoil of adolescence can be an exciting though difficult time. The new responsibilities of adulthood bring a vast array of challenges, experiences, and emotions.

The early stages of adulthood can be as confounding and groundbreaking as the years of adolescence. Decisions about work or university are often intermingled with the desire to travel or move away from home. There can be a great deal of pressure to appear mature and confident, and an individual still emerging from the experiences of adolescence may continue to feel slightly confused and overwhelmed. Many young adults feel that they are suddenly under an obligation to be responsible and organized, to have a sense of direction in life, and to assert independence that they still do not feel comfortable with. For this reason people commonly find this period somewhat disorienting and they frequently return to the family home. Much like a toddler, alternately exploring an environment, then checking for the presence of parents, a young adult may return to the family nest while still declaring his or her freedom.

COPING IN THE JOB MARKET

The psychoanalyst Sigmund Freud said that the two most important things in life are finding relationships that are intimate and gratifying and finding work that is fulfilling and challenging. Both of these prospects can seem daunting to a young person emerging from adolescence but still lacking in confidence and self-assurance. Self-fulfillment can often take a back seat to the fear of failure, the desire for financial reward, and the anxiety of not wanting to be left behind.

Many young adults still feel unsure about the career they wish to pursue and yet are conscious of the profound effect that work has on self-identity. One of the first questions that strangers ask each other when striking up a conversation is "What do you do?" because it reveals so much about personality and interests. However, it is worth remembering that many people experiment with a number of different careers before settling on a particular path. In 1994 researchers Susan Phillips and David Blustein found that nearly a third of people in their late twenties and early thirties had completely changed their career direction.

For some young people, getting their first job can be very difficult. Economic changes or layoffs in certain industries make it harder for inexperienced people to get work, and lengthy periods of unemployment are not uncommon. Unemployment often leads to personal feelings of dejection and a sense of exclusion from society. This in turn may cause depression or other mental or physical ill health.

One of the most difficult things to maintain during a period of unemployment is a feeling of self-worth and purpose. Having a range of interests, taking courses, and doing volunteer work can all help to keep spirits up and make constructive use of time until the right job becomes available.

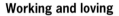

Working and loving
Finding the balance between a successful career and a happy relationship can be particularly difficult in early adulthood. The pressure to be successful and independent can lead to neglect of personal life. It is essential that you allow time for socializing and activities that you enjoy. Managing your time sensibly can help you work more efficiently, and developing a network of supportive relationships will help you through moments of stress.

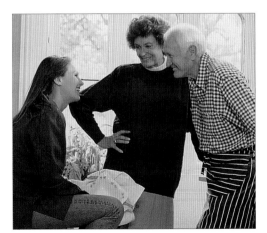

THE SUPPORTIVE FAMILY
The security and stability that come from having good family relationships are especially important in dealing successfully with the conflicting obligations of early adulthood.

CAREER DECISIONS

One of the greatest challenges of young adulthood can be finding a suitable career. After years of education, often pursuing a favorite subject, most individuals are confronted with a job market in which they have little experience and perhaps little interest. The desire to be financially independent can sometimes conflict with the wish to be fulfilled in your daily work. In choosing a career, think about the factors described below.

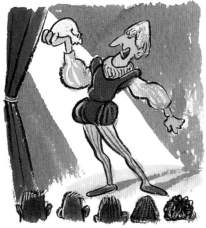

YOUR PERSONALITY
Consider the activities you enjoy and the skills they involve. Athletes often like working as part of a team, for example, while amateur actors may have a measure of creativity.

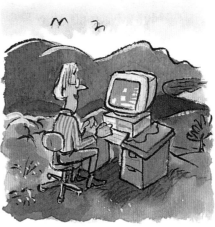

YOUR ENVIRONMENT
Think about the kind of place and the sort of people you want to be surrounded by. Investigate which careers offer the kind of working environment you want to be in.

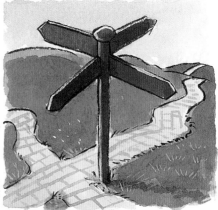

YOUR DIRECTION
Consider what you really want in terms of money and independence. How viable are your current aspirations, and will your chosen career path help you to reach them?

A NEW SET OF RELATIONSHIPS

While adolescent relationships tend to be based on sexual exploration or reassurance, most sexual relations in adulthood are focused on finding a partner. These experiences, which are generally more meaningful than teenage passions, can be both exciting and painful as the individual begins to learn more about himself or herself and the reality of the world. Close friendships are often at their most intense in these years as honesty, support, and intellectual stimulation take over the more superficial needs of simple socializing. It can be common for a person to develop close, nonsexual attachments to several persons because the need to belong and to feel secure overrides the common teenage desire to be independent. Many people find this is the first time they really come to understand their individuality.

COMMUNICATING

No matter what your age, the essence of a good relationship is always communication. Expressing anger, love, or fear enables a person to relieve mental anxieties and open up to another sympathetic individual. The true benefits of enjoying close, intimate relationships—whether with a sexual partner or a friend—depends on this ability to be as emotionally open and free as possible.

Expressing your unhappiness with a situation or person can be as emotionally positive as relating your joy, provided that the discussion is mutually constructive. This means respecting the other person's feelings while at the same time relieving personal anxiety and distress. Bridging a threatened gap is the only way to resolve personal fears of anger or rejection. By clearly communi-

DID YOU KNOW?
The number of single adult men and women is dramatically on the increase. In the past 30 years the marrying age has risen sharply, suggesting that adults are more concerned with establishing successful careers and independence before engaging in serious long-term relationships. In 1960 the average age of marriage was 23 for men and 20 for women; by 1994 it had risen to 27 for men and 25 for women.

cating your despair, frustration, or happiness, you enable a partner to understand how you feel and potentially bring about a greater sense of intimacy.

CONFLICT

There is no such thing as life without conflict, and whenever a person experiences an emotional struggle, there is a chance that this will be articulated externally. Young adulthood is usually the period in which many unresolved issues can become increasingly pressing and troublesome.

Work, personal relationships, responsibilities, and independence can all present a number of potentially conflicting situations. Suppressing or covering up the mental anxiety that such conflict causes, however, can often lead to distress and ill health. The wisest course is to express personal sentiment in a constructive and positive way. Withdrawing from conflict or evading an issue suggests that you feel a relationship may not be capable of withstanding or surviving the strains of confrontation. This lack of confidence can itself be destructive, and stagnation usually leads only to further personal frustration.

To keep yourself emotionally healthy, you need to keep your relationships in good condition. The open discussion of any conflict is a necessary part of this process, which also provides a good opportunity for developing your own self-awareness. Without conflict there would be no life, no energy, and no resolution. With each conflict that is successfully resolved, individuals realize that they can learn and survive together. Thinking of conflict as part of a natural human process will help to make it seem less frightening.

THE SINGLE LIFE

There is less pressure for an adult to marry and raise a family in today's society than existed a few years ago. Many people now accept that it is possible to be content and emotionally fulfilled without the social constraints of marriage or a partnership. The variety of relationships and experiences now open to an individual suggests that a person need not feel socially excluded or unusual because of a certainchoice of lifestyle or sexual orientation. However, a person's contentment with his or her situation depends

continued on page 46

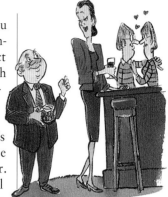

BIRDS OF A FEATHER
Despite the popular idea that opposites attract, statistics suggest that we tend to choose partners who are like ourselves. Even in terms of physical attractiveness, people usually date those whom they consider to be within their league. This reinforces self-confidence and reduces the likelihood of rejection.

RELEASE YOUR EMOTIONS

A number of therapies promote emotional well-being as well as physical relaxation through massage. One such therapy is Breema bodywork, based on old Kurdish practices that seek to relieve imbalances in the mind, body, and feelings. By activating self-corrective reflexes, the therapy rebalances body energies and improves clarity of mind. The "kidney charge" is a particularly good exercise for revitalizing energy flow.

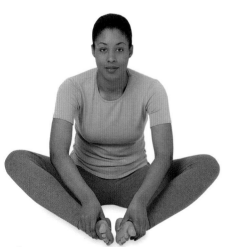

1 *Sit in a relaxed position and bring the soles of your feet together. Wrap your fingers over the tops of your feet with the thumbs pressing onto the balls.*

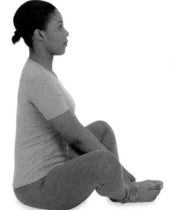

2 *Still holding your feet, straighten your arms as you stretch up and bring your spine into an erect position. Then gradually exhale, releasing the stretch and allowing your body to relax.*

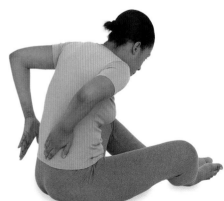

3 *Brush your hands up the inside of your legs and slide them to your back. Lean forward and slap the kidneys with alternating palms for three breaths. Finally, brush your hands down the legs to the starting position.*

Body Language

The spoken word is not the only way in which we communicate. Our gestures, facial expressions, and the way in which we hold our bodies all convey powerful messages to those around us and can have a strong impact on our relationships.

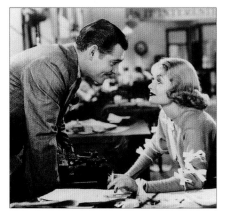

MUTUAL INTERACTION
Communication doesn't take place just with words. We talk and show our receptiveness to each other in bodily posture and interaction as well.

Understanding the impact of both our verbal and nonverbal speech can help us to improve communication with others. Learning to read and use body language can promote a better understanding of other people's feelings and help to avoid the frustrations of talking at cross-purposes. For example, we may unconsciously take up physical positions that are intimidating and make others feel inhibited or subordinate. Conversely, we may find it impossible to put across an opinion to an individual who physically shows an unwillingness to hear our point of view. Negative body language can lead to worsening patterns of communication that ultimately cause relationships to suffer and may eventually affect personal self-esteem.

THE IMPORTANCE OF EYE CONTACT

The ancient Roman orator Cicero said, "The face is the image of the soul." The human face is indeed capable of a remarkable subtlety of expression. A great deal of our everyday interaction with others is mediated through our faces and, more specifically, our eyes. An unblinking or intense gaze may be interpreted in conversation as insulting or threatening—an evolutionary throwback that can be seen in the behavior of other primates. However, no eye contact at all signals a lack of interest in the other person and is equally damaging to communication. Indeed, avoiding somebody's eyes is often seen as evidence of insincerity or dishonesty.

Eye contact is usually easiest when the orientation between individuals is indirect, giving the opportunity to break the gaze occasionally. Lowering your eyelids at the end of a sentence indicates to the other person that you are willing to hear his or her opinion,

and the same gesture performed while the other person is speaking indicates that you are prepared to concede a point. In fact, the area of a person's face at which you look during a discussion can convey a lot about your sincerity (see below). Looking at someone while that person is speaking sends the message that he or she has your attention—even though it is clearly

WHERE TO LOOK
The area of a person's face that you look at during interaction will convey a lot about how you feel. Gazing at different parts of the face suggests various levels of intimacy and seriousness.

not necessary to look at people in order to hear them. Avoiding the other person's gaze, however, may suggest you are trying to ignore what he or she is saying. Other affirmative gestures, like nodding, or nonverbal sounds of agreement are important for the same reason. Women tend to exhibit these gestures more often in conversation than men do, and this may partly explain why they are considered to be better listeners.

Looking at the triangle between a person's eyes and forehead will convey your seriousness.

Gazing at the area between the eyes and chin suggests social interaction.

The intimate gaze covers the whole area between the eyes and chest and suggests very personal interest.

OPENING UP YOUR BODY LANGUAGE

In the same way that certain phrases make another person feel defensive, so negative body language can elicit withdrawal or aggression. While attempts to communicate with an unresponsive partner can be frustrating, it is generally counter-productive to force an issue. Attempting to grab someone's attention physically or forcing him or her to confront you will only be seen as threatening. Standing directly in front of a person may be seen as an attack, especially if it is accompanied by a drastic reduction in the space between you. This may cause such protective gestures of closure as physical retreat, turning the back, flinching, or folding arms defensively.

Stance is also an important indication of intentions. Standing over someone indicates a desire to dominate the discussion and an unwillingness to allow an open expression of feelings. Conversely, taking up a physically laid-back posture if the other person is upright indicates lack of concern for the other's point of view and a feeling of superiority. The best approach is to match your stance to that of the other person as much as possible while remaining unthreatening. This indicates that you are willing to communicate as an equal.

When trying to reestablish some communication, the orientation of your body can also be important. Your body language should be direct and open; turning your body toward the other person but at a slightly oblique angle signals a wish to talk without forcing your presence aggressively. This positioning also facilitates eye contact and invites interaction. When coupled with some open-palmed hand gestures, which literally show that you have nothing to hide, this may help to establish trust between you and the other person.

As people pick up on your positive body language, their own bodies will open up. Studies show that those who are in agreement or have similar goals in a situation often mirror each other's body language.

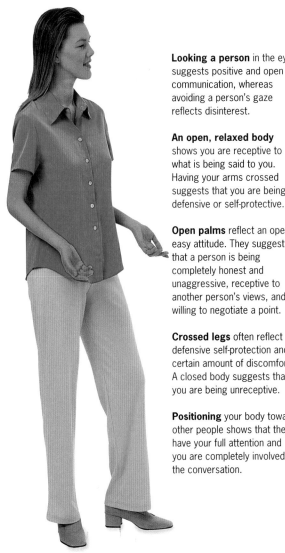

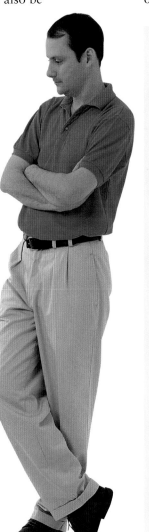

Looking a person in the eye suggests positive and open communication, whereas avoiding a person's gaze reflects disinterest.

An open, relaxed body shows you are receptive to what is being said to you. Having your arms crossed suggests that you are being defensive or self-protective.

Open palms reflect an open, easy attitude. They suggest that a person is being completely honest and unaggressive, receptive to another person's views, and willing to negotiate a point.

Crossed legs often reflect defensive self-protection and a certain amount of discomfort. A closed body suggests that you are being unreceptive.

Positioning your body toward other people shows that they have your full attention and you are completely involved in the conversation.

CONVERSATION ZONE

Opening the floor for discussion on an emotive topic is not always easy. It is especially hard when the other person involved is a close friend or partner. However, it is important not to assume that your feelings on a particular issue are obvious. Tackling the subject from a different angle should enable you to make your feelings clear and turn the situation into a positive one. For example, if you feel that your partner is avoiding conversation by watching television, do not criticize him or her. Understand that there may be a reason for this behavior—preoccupation or fatigue, for example—but explain calmly that this makes you feel rejected. This approach should help your partner understand the emotional impact of his or her actions. Being unable to deny or reject your personal feelings, he or she is likely to be more receptive to your comments.

CHILDLESSNESS

Coping with childlessness can be emotionally traumatic for a couple. Their own desire to raise a family can be exacerbated by social pressures to produce children and, very often, the success of their friends and peers at producing families.

Personal disappointment and anxiety may turn to acute grief and anger, especially if a couple is unable to discuss their emotions openly. Stress can then further inhibit a woman's chances of conception. Many couples find that seeking both psychological and physical help is the only way to deal with the frustration and to prevent the distress from damaging their relationship.

Even deciding not to have children can have its own emotional impact. Although increasingly many couples are remaining childless through choice, they still experience a certain amount of social pressure to conform and raise a family. Their parents often express a desire for grandchildren, while friends with families may repeatedly comment on the rewards of parenthood. In dealing with such comments and criticisms, a couple should try to remember that having a family is their own choice. If your own personal circumstances, ambitions, beliefs, or preferences lead you not to want children, try not to be affected by social pressure.

THE BABY BLUES
Many women experience the "baby blues," a form of depression, shortly after giving birth as excitement is replaced by exhaustion and anxiety. If you or your partner feel that things are becoming overwhelming, do not think that seeking help is an admission of failure. It is in the whole family's interest to make the mother—and the newborn—as happy and emotionally secure as possible.

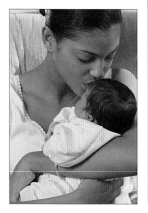

not just on individual personality but also on social acceptability. We derive much of our sense of security from social reinforcement, and many people feel that they are being wrongly judged or criticized for their marriage or partnership decisions.

Although many individuals feel personally happy with being single, their awareness of friends marrying or settling down can bring a sense of insecurity. It is common for people in their late twenties and thirties to suddenly become aware of their age and feel that some biological clock is ticking away, gradually reducing the time they have in which to find a partner or consider having a family. If a person is not single by choice, this mental awareness can cause even greater anxiety and apprehension. One of the hardest emotional experiences during this period of life can be trading off independence and freedom with the restrictions and intimacy of a close relationship.

PARENTHOOD
No matter how planned or anticipated a baby may be, becoming a parent can create emotional turmoil. The challenge of having your life turned upside down, of being responsible for a baby's helpless needs, can be both incredibly frightening and fulfilling. The fact that being a parent is so common does not make the experience any less unnerving. The sudden shock of devoting your life to another can elicit all kinds of unexpected feelings, including jealousy and

resentment, as well as bewilderment over your own identity and feelings of maturity. Many people find it difficult to reconcile their experiences as an independent person with having to take responsibility for another, completely dependent individual.

New parents often acquire new insight into their relationships with their own parents. Many people claim to feel an increased sense of respect and understanding for their parents as they come to terms with their new parenthood roles.

Grandparents can be a great help in bringing up children, although they can also be a source of family conflict. Much of your attitude will depend on how good you feel about your own childhood and whether you agree with the ideas on care and discipline held by your own or your spouse's parents. While all parents want to feel that they can cope on their own, accepting the good advice and experience of others can often be of immense help. Supportive family structures, with good relationships at all levels, will help provide the best possible security for your children.

Although parenthood is undeniably hard work, the majority of parents believe that the anxieties and stress are far outweighed by the rewards and happiness that having children can bring. If you take time to consider your own apprehensions and limitations before undertaking such responsibility, the role of a parent can herald a whole series of new and fulfilling adult experiences.

MATURITY AND THE MIDDLE YEARS

Although most people feel relatively settled in their middle years, the period can still be one of transition. The insecurities of youth make way for the emotional realities of a changing lifestyle.

Throughout life we are constantly changing our perception of ourselves and other people. When you are a young adult, you may imagine that you will feel emotionally secure and confident by the time you reach midlife, but the reality is that most people still feel they are developing mentally and emotionally and adapting to change in this period. People with families see their children grow up and move on, while the responsibility for older relatives often becomes more intense. In this age-conscious culture, growing up is seen as positive but growing older tends to be viewed in a negative light, and this view can affect a person's esteem and self-perception.

The term "midlife crisis" reflects the common anxieties, even bewilderment, that growing older can bring about. Denying yourself these emotions or allowing yourself to become depressed about them will intensify your internal conflict even further. Accepting these life changes and progressing through them can lead to a deeper sense of self-awareness and the opportunity to feel more complete and whole.

FAMILY ADJUSTMENT

The crises of most middle-aged people center around feelings of loss. While some of these losses are real and tangible, it is not uncommon for people to feel that they are losing a sense of self and subsequently suffer a crisis of identity. Adjusting to the loss of a parent or the independence of a son or daughter can evoke strong feelings of disorientation and ineptitude. The sudden freedom from parental responsibility can often leave an individual with a lack of direction and a sense of pointlessness—rather than optimistic feelings of more freedom and opportunity. For couples such changes can precipitate a crisis in their relationship. If you are mentally unprepared to make adjustments or are unable to discuss your fears and anxieties, personal apprehensions may become a source of conflict. Couples who are prepared to rediscover each other as individuals are better able to face the reality of advancing age and accept and enjoy the changes that it brings.

TAOISM AND LONGEVITY

Many Taoist philosophers have asserted that the natural human life span is at least 100 years. In order to reach this age, they recommend that individuals strive for a balanced life, combining a calm, moderate pace with regular breathing and exercise routines and avoiding extreme emotions. Doing the two Taoist exercises below every day is said to increase longevity by improving circulation and energy flow. It may also inhibit wrinkles.

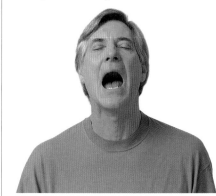 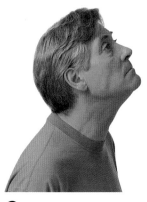

1 *Tilt your head back slightly, eyes closed, and open your mouth wide as if yawning deeply. Then open your eyes and contort your facial muscles into a grimace. Repeat these exercises several times each day.*

2 *Tilt your head back and jut out your chin as far as it will go. Hold the stretch for about 1 minute, then relax the muscles. Repeat the exercise two more times.*

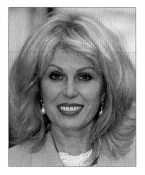

LIFE BEGINS AT 40
While some people reach their middle years and resign themselves to a life without much challenge or excitement, others take the opportunity to reinvent themselves and grab a second chance. The famous British actress Joanna Lumley is a classic example of somebody who seized new opportunities in her career that took her from 1970s fame in The New Avengers *to the outrageous role of Patsy in the 1990s hit comedy* Absolutely Fabulous.

PHYSICAL ADJUSTMENT

Just as adolescence brings about obvious physical change, middle age brings with it some bodily alterations as well. Adjusting to a less active metabolism and possibly developing some physical infirmities can be difficult for an individual who has always enjoyed a healthy, active lifestyle. Nevertheless, there is no reason that a person shouldn't be as physically and emotionally well in mid life as in younger adulthood.

As people grow older, it becomes increasingly important that they take good care of their bodies. Making sure that your diet is healthy and well balanced and getting regular exercise can help ensure that you remain as physically fit, healthy, and attractive as you ever were.

The secret of adjusting to physical change is to accept rather than hide from reality. Successfully adapting your clothes, hairstyle, and general outlook to enhance your physical appearance can not only keep you attractive but also boost self-confidence. As a result, you should feel as emotionally complete and vital as you did in your late teens or twenties because you still have control over how you look and feel.

NUTRITIONAL HEAVY WEIGHTS

Eating healthfully can slow down many of the aging processes and reduce the risks of developing serious illness. Taking good care of your body is a way of confirming that you deserve good health and a full and energetic life. A few changes to your diet can reap impressive results by making you feel and look better, boost your energy levels, and help you to feel self-confident. Except for sweets, most foods provide a range of useful vitamins and minerals, but the four described below are particularly beneficial for maintaining a healthy immune system and tackling the physical effects of middle age. Not only should you include them in your daily diet but you should select as wide a variety of them as possible for optimum benefit. Regularly trying new fruits, vegetables, and grains rewards your taste buds too.

WHOLE GRAINS

Whole-grain breads and other grain products are excellent sources of complex carbohydrates, iron, and the B vitamins—all of which are necessary for maintaining energy. They also contain good amounts of fiber, needed for regularity.

FRUITS

Fruits of every type offer many nutritional benefits. Some are high in vitamin C, others in vitamin A, and all are rich in bioflavonoids; all of the above are antioxidants that help protect against disease. People who eat two to four servings of fruit a day have a lower risk for heart disease, stroke, and some types of cancer.

GREEN VEGETABLES

Vegetables with dark green leaves, especially the crucifers such as broccoli and kale, are good sources of antioxidants and phytochemicals,.which help fight the aging process and may reduce the risk of certain cancers. They also provide insoluble fiber, which supports regularity.

COLD-WATER FISH

Oily. or cold-water, fish, such as sardines, mackerel, and salmon, are excellent sources of the omega-3 fatty acids, which have been shown to reduce the risk of heart disease and stroke when eaten twice a week. Flaxseeds and flax-seed oil are good plant sources of the omega-3 fats.

A Communication Problem

Midlife changes often take their toll on relationships. As people start to reassess themselves as individuals, they may also begin to reevaluate their family lives and yearn for further change. Not discussing these changes and feelings can make problems worse and cause a couple to question each other's behavior and attitudes.

Sue and Robert have been married for 30 years and have two grown sons. They have enjoyed a happy marriage and family life but, now that the boys have moved away, Sue would like to go back to work and begin a new life. She is taking computer courses but is discouraged about the lack of jobs for someone her age. She also feels that Robert doesn't really have any interest in her attempts at a new career and that he is not being very supportive of her efforts.

Robert is sympathetic with Sue's frustration but feels that his own needs require more attention. He is under intense pressure at work and believes that, despite all of the long hours he puts in, Sue does not appreciate how important his job is.

WHAT SHOULD SUE AND ROBERT DO?

The longer Sue and Robert do not discuss what is happening in their relationship, the more likely it is that they will proceed down the slippery slope of marital breakdown. Because there are deep and powerful emotions at play, it is important that Sue and Robert begin by taking small steps in communicating with each other—one marathon session of opening everything up may do little except cause more anger and pain.

Setting aside a definite time for discussion each week and taking turns listening to each other talk about their feelings, will help both of them adjust better to the changes going on in their lives and to understand each others' anxieties.

EMOTIONAL HEALTH
Emotional and physical stress can cause people to be less patient in listening to each other's problems.

WORK
If work is allowed to take over your life, it can be very difficult to make time for other things. Not discussing your frustrations only adds further to stress.

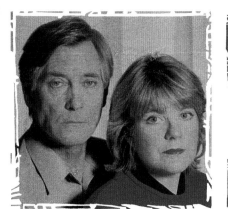

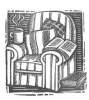

LIFESTYLE
A change in family setup can be very disorienting and add to emotional insecurity.

Action Plan

EMOTIONAL HEALTH
Relieve pressures by opening up and talking to each other about feelings and problems. Make more time for regular communication throughout the week.

WORK
Recognize the importance of work and find ways to support each other's career needs.

LIFESTYLE
Set aside at least one evening a week to enjoy an activity together. Perhaps taking up a new hobby will provide a good opportunity to meet other like-minded people.

HOW THINGS TURNED OUT FOR SUE AND ROBERT

With patience and a desire to make things work, Robert and Sue began to talk to each other about their feelings. It was difficult at the beginning, but they now accept that they both have unfulfilled needs and are missing the family life that they used to enjoy. They agreed to make an effort to go out at least once a week and adjust to their new way of life by socializing more with other people. Sue plans to begin looking for work soon.

A THERAPY FOR REDUCING INHIBITIONS

A common source of confusion for people in their middle years comes from a sense of inhibition, of being unable to embrace change because of insecurity and lack of confidence. Many therapists believe that we simply grit our teeth and carry on, trying to protect ourselves from our true emotions.

Watsu is a type of water therapy that aims to reconcile these inner conflicts. It involves sessions of massage and body manipulation while floating in a pool of warm water. The relaxing, liberating water enables the therapist to manipulate the vertebrae of the spine, stretching and moving the body to increase its flexibility. The mental and physical freedom that Watsu fosters allows a patient to relax completely and release emotional anguish. For many people the womb-like state enables a return to the freedom of infancy.

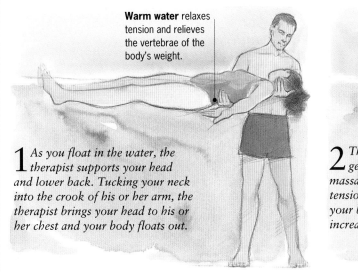

Warm water relaxes tension and relieves the vertebrae of the body's weight.

1 *As you float in the water, the therapist supports your head and lower back. Tucking your neck into the crook of his or her arm, the therapist brings your head to his or her chest and your body floats out.*

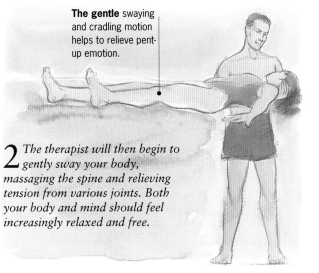

The gentle swaying and cradling motion helps to relieve pent-up emotion.

2 *The therapist will then begin to gently sway your body, massaging the spine and relieving tension from various joints. Both your body and mind should feel increasingly relaxed and free.*

CAREER ADJUSTMENT

Your career and working life may also become an issue during this period. People often feel stuck on one career path or at a certain level of responsibility and see little possibility to make a change. There may be a sense of life closing in as financial issues and the force of habit reduce a person's sense of options. In many respects the feeling of being stuck relates more to attitude and outlook than to reality. If you are unhappy in your career, financial considerations may not necessarily be a restriction. You may be more financially secure than you realize, with a mortgage nearly paid off and major household items purchased. With careful planning, returning to full-time study or retraining in another career field could well be manageable.

In fact, it is often subconscious anxiety and a lack of self-confidence rather than practical restrictions that make changes in lifestyle seem so difficult. Chapter 6 examines a number of therapies that explore how personal reluctance and inhibition may be preventing us from leading more successful and fulfilling and happier lives.

JUNG'S MERITS OF MIDDLE AGE

Contrary to most Western ideas on aging, the psychiatrist Carl Jung proposed that it is from midlife onward that an individual truly achieves his or her potential. While Sigmund Freud believed that the greatest amount of character formation occurs in infancy, Jung claimed that midlife is a crucial turning point that enables an individual to take up new opportunities. He pointed out that physical, intellectual, and social developments occur at different times, so while a body may be physically less capable in older age, mental experience may help increase spiritual growth. For this reason Jung believed that people actually have the potential to enjoy life *more* as they grow older.

Jung argued that the inner changes that affect a person in later life provide scope for setting new goals. The increased focus on the self can lead to heightened self-awareness, fostering creative impulses and, quite literally, a new lease on life. Similarly, confronting negative aspects of the self provides an opportunity for reevaluation. Put simply, later ages have as much to offer in terms of personal development as youth.

OLD AGE

Although it still requires adjustment to accept some limitations, old age can be one of the most secure periods of life. Many oldsters enjoy new opportunities and the rewards of maturity.

Some people fear the approach of old age as heralding the end of life's prime—indeed, the end of life itself. This predominantly Western belief tends to equate increasing years with futility, as if an older person were no longer able to make a useful contribution to society and had to become a burden on everybody else. The truth is, however, that better living standards and medical care mean that more and more people are enjoying a long, healthy, and fit old age and continuing to contribute to the well-being of those around them.

ADAPTING EMOTIONALLY

There can be little doubt that the body declines physically with advancing age. Although efforts to maintain personal health and fitness can help slow down some of the changes, weakening muscles and joints, together with slower body responses, are generally inevitable—and can be frustrating to the person who feels as mentally active and alert as ever.

Adapting to the physical realities of old age can be one of the biggest emotional challenges facing an older person. The fact that you are not as physically as able as you once were can lead to depression and a lack of self-esteem, which may then affect your health and ability to take care of yourself. Some older people actually stop looking after themselves, developing a kind of paranoia about their declining abilities and, in effect, deciding to give up. Although medication can help relieve this kind of depression, making an effort to keep a strong grip on reality is equally important. Allowing yourself to become increasingly depressed will only intensify feelings of loneliness and futility. On the other hand, if you consider all the experience and knowledge that you have to offer, you can enjoy the fruits of your efforts throughout life. Rather than old age being a period of winding down, it can offer the advantages of seniority and more freedom to socialize and relax.

ADJUSTING TO RETIREMENT

Retirement can be a time of great opportunity for you to realize long-held dreams and ambitions. After a lifetime of family and work commitments, retirement heralds the opportunity to spend some time on yourself, fulfilling personal aspirations and enjoying a newfound sense of freedom. In order to reap the full benefits, however, you must realize that retirement requires a certain amount of mental preparation. You may need to restructure part of your life and be prepared to socialize in different circles and develop new friends. Exploring and taking up new activities can make the transition easier and can be a good way to meet like-minded individuals. Some people treat retirement more as an opportunity for a career change. Writing a novel, for example,

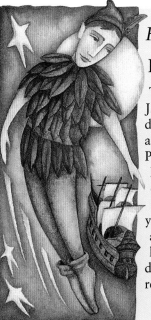

Fables and myths

PETER PAN

The character Peter Pan, created by J. M. Barrie in 1904, is famous for his decision never to grow up. After many adventures with his childhood friends, Peter decides to stay in Never Never Land rather than return to the realities of human existence. Peter Pan embodies the wish of many people to stay forever young and avoid the responsibilities of adulthood. The name of his retreat, however, illustrates the fact that his dream is impossible to achieve; it must remain a romantic ideal.

MEMORY AND OLD AGE

Many people in their older years become frustrated at what seems to be failing memory. Although the coordination between short- and long-term memory does deteriorate with age, this does not mean that experiences and knowledge are forgotten forever. Most people find that even though they cannot remember as many things as they would like to, when they do retrieve an event from the past, they remember it with great detail and clarity.

and becoming involved in community issues are excellent ways of keeping the mind as alert and active as ever. Ultimately, you can be as busy and on the go as you want to be.

COPING WITH LOSS

It is a sad fact that old age tends to bring the highest number of personal losses—both in terms of ability and close relationships. Losing a partner or spouse is considered to be the most traumatic experience of this period, and its effects are both physical and psychological. Many people react so badly that they suffer their own subsequent illnesses or fall into serious depression and self-neglect. Anybody in this position needs

SUPREME AGILITY
Many older people retain physical independence by keeping fit and prove that it is possible to maintain excellent fitness levels throughout life. At various competitions supremely fit senior citizens demonstrate their agility and determination.

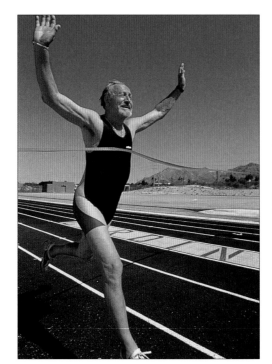

emotional and medical support in order to come to terms with the new circumstances. Reassessing yourself as a worthwhile individual means accepting this enforced independence and finding the will and strength to continue life alone.

Losing friends and family members can also make individuals increasingly aware of their own mortality. Overcoming the personal loss and loneliness is made harder by the reality that old age provides fewer opportunities for fresh starts. As with any other stage in life, deciding how you will embrace these changes largely determines how they will eventually affect you.

Although nobody relishes the thought of having to adapt to circumstances beyond his or her personal control, taking on new challenges can be enormously stimulating. Old age offers as many opportunities for new experiences as any other stage of life. In fact, it arguably offers more because of the increased freedom provided by retirement, but only if each new challenge is approached with an open mind. If you can be positive and discuss your fears and anxieties without dwelling on them, you will stand a better chance of recovering from setbacks and going on to enjoy a series of new, exciting, and different experiences.

DEPENDENCY

Becoming dependent on other people for the basic necessities of life is a common and understandable fear for most older people. Having to rely on others can undermine a person's self-confidence and increase feelings of frustration and encumbrance. The freedom of independence is difficult to give up, and some older persons channel their resentment into demanding cantankerousness. Furthermore, people who refuse to admit their need for practical help may cause themselves further harm. While insisting on

DID YOU KNOW?
Although the moment of death appears to be beyond our control, some researchers believe that this is not entirely the case. For example, the deaths of old people have been shown to be highest in the period immediately following their birthdays, which suggests that some can will themselves to stay alive for important events.

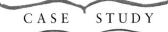

Increasing Spirituality

The elderly often find themselves bereft of the things that are generally taken for granted, including good health, physical and mental agility, and intimate relationships. How each person copes with such losses will vary, but many individuals find that an increasing awareness of their own and universal spirituality can be a great source of comfort.

Albert is a 78-year-old widower whose wife died five years ago and whose two sons now work in other states, so he sees them infrequently. Although Albert still lives in the same house he and his wife bought 40 years ago, all of his close friends have either died or moved away. Most of Albert's neighbors are now young families who are busily involved with their own lives. Although there are clubs he could join, Albert feels that he needs something more meaningful and personally rewarding. He has an urge to better understand the experiences of his life and find what seems to be the missing piece. Albert remains outwardly as cheerful as possible, but he feels that his life has lost some of its meaning.

WHAT SHOULD ALBERT DO?

Many older people seek deeper spirituality and the meaning of life because they find it fulfilling and a change from the realities of the daily world. Joining a worship or meditation group would introduce Albert to other seekers and provide opportunities for new experiences. Such a group can also be a source of new friendships.

Albert should reflect on what would bring him comfort and perhaps explore both Eastern and Western philosophies to find what would suit him best. Learning about other religions and cultures might help him gain a better perspective on the experiences of his life and enable him to face the future with more optimism and direction.

Action Plan

LIFESTYLE
Find a worship or other spiritually motivated group in order to come to a better understanding of life experiences and make contact with like-minded people.

FAMILY
Maintain as much contact with the family as possible. Phone and write regularly and try to see them at least once a year.

EMOTIONAL HEALTH
Using meditation, prayer, and/or relaxation techniques, explore ways to relieve emotional anxieties and deal with fear.

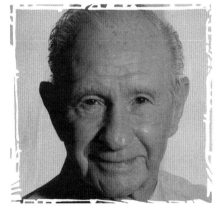

LIFESTYLE
Accepting and adapting to change can get harder with increasing age.

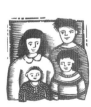

FAMILY
Maintaining closeness with family members over a long distance can be difficult.

EMOTIONAL HEALTH
Looking back over your life can be both enlightening and bewildering.

HOW THINGS TURNED OUT FOR ALBERT

Albert became very interested in Jungian theories on old age and started to attend meetings where people discussed both psychology and spirituality. He learned meditation techniques, which have helped him to relax and feel more complete within himself, but the classes have also provided him with greater self-confidence. Albert has now made several new friends of all ages and feels that he is a valuable contributor to and member of the group.

ENJOYING OLD AGE
One of the greatest pleasures of later life is enjoying the companionship of your family.

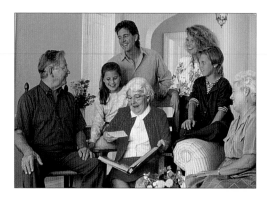

their ability to look after themselves, elderly people can easily forget to eat or lock the door, for example. Through a reluctance to admit their needs, they not only place their own physical health in jeopardy but also lay further worry and responsibility on younger family members, who may find it difficult to balance their relative's desire for independence with safety.

Overcoming such pride and stubborn self-denial is another necessary stage for mental well-being. Accepting your new, more dependent identity in old age is as important to good psychological health as is coming to terms with your adolescent or middle-aged self. This stage of development needs as much adjustment and understanding as any other period in your life. By acknowledging

their internal and physical changes, many older people go on to experience a very deep level of consciousness and find solace in a new sense of self and spirituality.

SPIRITUALITY AND SOLITUDE

For many older people the loss of physical and even mental strength often coincides with a search for inner peace. In coming to accept that death is inevitable, some individuals find a greater degree of spirituality, becoming increasingly detached and philosophical about their physical and emotional life experiences. This optimistic overview is often not given much attention in modern society, but its significance to individuals can be paramount.

The capacity not only to be alone but also to enjoy solitude is particularly important for a person in old age, when there may be a loss of external support. While loneliness involves a painful awareness of the absence of others, solitude reflects a sense of comfort, awareness, and acceptance. In facing and accepting death, older people learn to acknowledge that they both came into and will leave the world in solitude. Either through conventional religion or a self-developed philosophy, they can achieve a calm, detached inner peace.

THE FOUR STAGES OF BEREAVEMENT

Coming to terms with the death of somebody close to you can be a long and difficult process. It is normal for people to lose friends or members of their family throughout life, but during the later years many have to undergo the turmoil repeatedly. Research

conducted in 1990 suggests that every individual goes through a series of reactions when experiencing grief. Although each person will vary in response and cope differently, most people will have to work through all of the stages for full recovery.

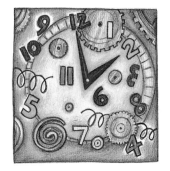

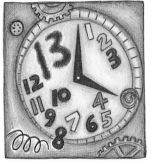

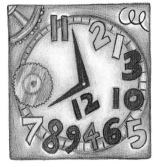

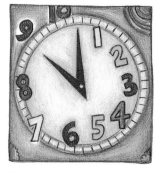

The first stage is shock and involves a profound sense of disbelief and numbness. The apparent unreality of the situation can last for a few hours or for several days.

The second stage includes psychological protest. An individual yearns for the deceased person and may hallucinate or fantasize that he or she has actually seen the person being mourned.

The third stage involves a feeling of disorganization and despair because life feels overwhelming without the deceased person. This period often lasts for a long time, running into months or years.

The final stage is one of detachment. Although the deceased is not forgotten, the grieving individual begins to reorganize his or her life, regaining a sense of purpose and establishing new roles.

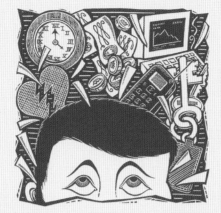

CHAPTER 3

THE POWER OF THE MIND

The way in which we think and process information can affect the way we feel. Our thought patterns can therefore have a significant bearing on our emotional, mental, and physical well-being. This chapter looks at how to recognize when we are falling into negative thought patterns and how we can influence our cognitive processes in order to raise our self-esteem and enjoy life more.

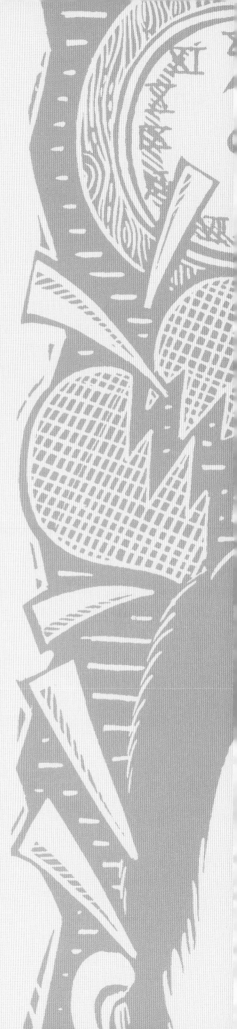

THE MIND AND HEALTH CONNECTION

The effects of emotions and thought processes are not confined to your mind; they can extend to every part of your body, triggering physical changes and affecting your health.

Mind over body
Some people think that doctors are skeptical about the power of the mind to influence the course of an illness. However, a 1996 report by the American Academy of Family Physicians showed that over 75 percent of its members believe that a patient's prayers can aid in recovery from illness.

When you experience a strong emotion, your body responds with certain physical reactions. For example, if you become anxious, the symptoms you experience signify that your body is physically preparing to cope with a threatening situation (see page 20). After the sense of danger has passed, the response to the stress should quickly subside and your body return to its normal condition. Longer-lasting emotions, such as continuous anxiety or suppressed anger, tend to keep low levels of physical response simmering. This can lead eventually to physical

THE AUTONOMIC NERVOUS SYSTEM

The two-part autonomic nervous system connects internal organs, glands, and involuntary muscles to the central nervous system. It regulates heartbeat, breathing, and digestion and is responsible for helping your body react to emotion. Sweaty palms, increased pulse, and rapid breathing in a moment of anxiety are all brought on by the part called the sympathetic nervous system as it prepares the body for "fight or flight." The second, or parasympathetic, nervous system works in reverse, gradually calming you down after an emergency and returning the body to normal. By slowing down your breathing and restimulating digestion, the system helps you relax again and restore balance.

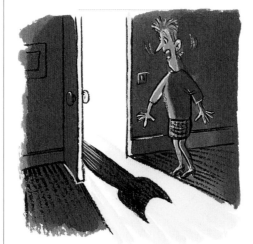

SYMPATHETIC NERVOUS SYSTEM (SNS)
Preparing the body for using energy, the SNS accelerates breathing and heartbeat, inhibits the salivary glands, releases glucose from the liver, and relaxes the bladder.

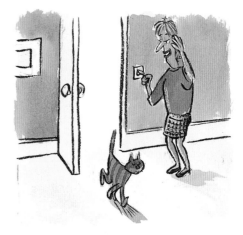

PARASYMPATHETIC NERVOUS SYSTEM (PNS)
Stimulating those processes that conserve the body's energy, the PNS decelerates breathing and heartbeat, stimulates the salivary glands, and contracts the bladder.

THINKING YOURSELF ILL

In most people the mind and body work together in harmony and maintain a workable balance. If the mind begins to overpower or misinterpret the body's signals, however, a person can begin to panic about his or her health and make anxious, irrational judgments.

Hypochondriasis is a condition in which a person fears becoming critically ill and interprets minor aches and pains as signs of more serious conditions. A hypochondriac might interpret a slight twinge in the chest, for example, as an impending heart attack or lie awake night after night worrying about cancer. While people should be alert to their physical well-being, obsession over symptoms can be debilitating. And excessive anxiety about health may actually inhibit the immune system.

these people tended to seek out challenging and stressful work and frequently suppressed their emotions.

Labeled the Type A behavior pattern, these characteristics incline a person to accumulate stress and subsequently increase the risk of suffering from heart conditions. Because of these distinct emotional reactions, the bodies of Type A individuals are often subject to higher blood pressure and an increased pulse rate, which if maintained for prolonged periods can produce excessive wear on arteries. At the same time, their increased levels of adrenaline, the hormone used by the body in times of stress, can lead to fatty deposits on the walls of their blood vessels. Both of these conditions are factors in cardiovascular disease.

Even the characteristic ways in which you stand or sit can affect your health. If you are naturally tense in your posture, this self-protective stance can lead to aches in the back and shoulders, constricted joints, and tightened muscles. Similarly, if you feel like a victim or are overpowered by events, it is quite possible that you have a "collapsed posture," in which the spine is stooped and weak, causing the shoulders to slump forward and the chest to be constricted.

Although we all adopt different positions occasionally, prolonged holding of a posture that restricts the body's movement or inhibits muscular action or breathing will take a toll on health. Aches, pains, and muscle strain can become more serious conditions in which the body fails to function at its optimum and other organs and joints are stressed unnecessarily. Tension headaches, stomach ulcers, and inefficient breathing are all examples of conditions that can be caused or worsened by anxious posture. It seems that a person's characteristic way of dealing with problems and expressing emotions can actually help to determine how healthy his or her body will be.

PSYCHOSOMATIC ILLNESS

A psychosomatic illness is a condition that is caused or intensified by a person's emotional problems. Despite a common perception to the contrary, the illness and its symptoms are not imaginary but very real manifestations of pain. They can range from the relatively trivial, such as tension headaches, to more serious conditions, such as heart problems and even blindness or

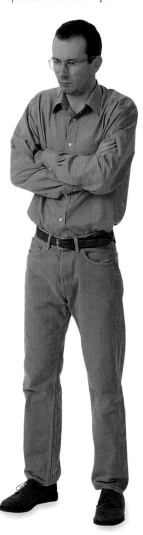

A TENSE BODY
People who are naturally tense often reflect their pent-up emotion in their posture—through a tightened rib cage, shortened neck, or rounded shoulders—any of which can cause pain.

distress and a reduction in the effectiveness of the immune system, making you more vulnerable to infections and general illness. Hypertension, which is often associated with emotional stress, can cause damage to the entire circulatory system if it is allowed to continue for prolonged periods of time.

PERSONALITY AND ILLNESS

There is increasing evidence that a person's character and attitude can help determine the effects that illness will have. We all know people who overdramatize every ailment, who have headaches worse than anyone else's or retire to bed at the first sign of a cold. Conversely, many other people tend to carry on in spite of ill health, disability, or pronounced pain, continuing to work and to pursue a normal life. Some of them even claim to fight off ill health by exerting mind over matter.

Although the way in which individuals deal with their suffering is largely a personal matter, scientists do believe that people can vary in their vulnerability to illness depending on their personality. Research carried out by three American physicians in 1979 showed that many patients who had suffered heart attacks shared certain personality traits. Often competitive and impatient, paralysis. The point at which the mind becomes responsible for these very real physical symptoms is difficult to determine.

How psychosomatic illness occurs

Most people experience minor psychosomatic symptoms, such as nervousness or anxiety, from time to time. These sensations may be brought on by any big or new experience that challenges emotional balance. The excitement and anxiety of starting a new job, getting married, or speaking in public can bring on a variety of symptoms, including headache, dizziness, indigestion, and diarrhea. Even yearning to have children or experiencing the excitement of becoming a parent can cause some people to develop psychosomatic symptoms.

Intense and prolonged stress can trigger serious physical disorders, such as eczema, psoriasis, ulcers, and high blood pressure. In most cases medical treatment can help to clear up the symptoms, but it cannot address the cause of the problem. Sufferers need to reassess their lifestyle and consider the possibility that emotional influences may be prolonging their illness and that these need to be addressed in order for recovery to be complete.

Many psychiatrists believe that prolonged psychosomatic illness derives from an inability to deal with normal emotions. People who suppress or fail to understand their anxiety, anger, or grief, for example, may discover that these feelings become expressed in other ways, including physical ones. While people who recognize that they are absorbing unhealthy stress may identify the connection and do something to coun-

REDUCING INHIBITION
Therapies for psycho-somatic illness often focus on reducing inhibitions and encouraging people to communicate by touch.

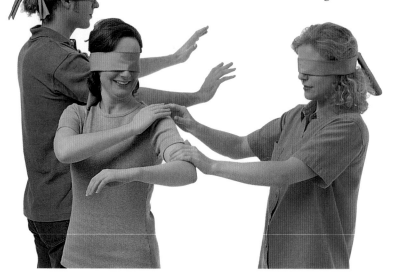

DID YOU KNOW?
Queen Mary I of England was so desperate to have a child that she experienced a "phantom pregnancy." In the autumn of 1554, convinced that she was pregnant, the queen developed many of the physical symptoms, including a swollen abdomen, milk production, and even sensations of a baby's movement inside her. Nine months later, however, no baby arrived. All her symptoms eventually disappeared.

teract it, others may subconsciously believe that emotional expression is wrong. This erroneous belief can lead to a buildup of pain and anger that will release themselves in physical symptoms while the sufferer continues to think that he or she has picked up a virus or other ailment.

Dealing with psychosomatic illness

When you experience any illness other than a minor, short-lived complaint, you should consult your doctor. If you suspect that the problem might have an emotional cause or that your emotional state might be making it worse, try to give the doctor as complete a picture as possible. Conversely, if you think that the illness is purely physical, don't take offense if the doctor suggests an emotional link. Psychosomatic illnesses are nothing to be ashamed of, and almost everybody develops them to varying degrees at some point in their lives. Whatever the doctor's diagnosis, the first step is to cure the physical symptoms and then to tackle the psychological ones.

Many therapies for dealing with psychosomatic illness focus on helping people to express their emotions. This can be a very difficult process because people have built up such effective control mechanisms over their feelings. In encounter groups members are encouraged to share their problems and feelings, sometimes by shouting, crying, or touching one another. Much of the therapy focuses on reducing inhibitions, so warm-up exercises designed to break down natural restraints on behavior are important. Members might be asked to blindfold themselves and walk around the room with their hands outstretched, communicating only by touch. Or they may work together to carry another member around the room.

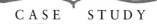

A Psychosomatic Sufferer

Being unable to express your emotions can cause them to become bottled up inside and gnaw away at you on a subconscious level. This process can eventually lead to debilitating physical symptoms that make daily life harder to cope with. Accepting that your physical complaint may have an emotional cause can be a prerequisite to feeling better.

Roy, 42, is a human resources manager at a merchant bank. He was only 12 when his mother died of cancer and he was left to look after his younger brothers while his father worked. In order to cope with the demands of this role, Roy set aside his own emotional needs and concentrated on meeting the demands of others.

Roy has always projected the image of someone who does not need emotional support from other people. Since recently being turned down for a promotion that he dearly wanted, however, he has felt dejected and depressed. Normally not prone to illness, Roy has developed pains in his stomach. His doctor has diagnosed an ulcer that he believes is stress related.

WHAT SHOULD ROY DO?

Roy has caused himself an immense amount of stress and pain by bottling up the hurt and rejection he felt when he wasn't promoted. He has learned to avoid expressing emotion, and now this unacknowledged pain is releasing itself in physical illness. He needs to become less emotionally inhibited if he wants to prevent a similar problem from happening again in the future.

If Roy can learn to admit that he has emotional needs, he will be better able to talk through his feelings with friends and colleagues. Coming to terms with the emotions of his childhood, perhaps through group therapy, might enable Roy to vent some of the anger and pain that have been building up inside.

Action Plan

HEALTH
Medical treatment can relieve physical symptoms, but emotional problems have to be resolved in order to get at the cause.

EMOTIONAL HEALTH
It's necessary to accept that there is little point in being emotionally unmoved. Failing to express and share feelings can lead to further emotional and physical turmoil.

WORK
Try to keep a sense of proportion at work and do not let problems or disappointments take over your emotional life.

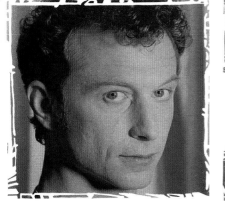

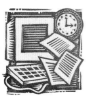

WORK
Problems and disappointments at work can be a major cause of stress.

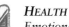

HEALTH
Emotional problems can cause physical illness, and hiding problems from yourself and others will not prevent this.

EMOTIONAL HEALTH
When emotions are strongly felt, you cannot make them go away by ignoring or denying them—they will nag away in your subconscious mind.

HOW THINGS TURNED OUT FOR ROY

Roy's doctor provided medication for the ulcer, but he also encouraged Roy to look closely at his attitude toward coping with disappointment. Roy started to attend a self-help group and gradually gained the confidence to talk about his feelings. After a while, Roy felt able to discuss things with close friends. Their helpful and supportive reaction has enabled him to become much more open emotionally and ready to ask for help.

Thoughts, memory, and feelings

Some mental health experts believe that you can use your rational mind to challenge negative memories, emotions, and behavior and live a more healthful, balanced life.

Just as negative emotions can produce harmful physical effects, so can positive emotions and attitudes provide health benefits. There is increasing evidence that people with a positive outlook are healthier than those who are prone to negativity and pessimism. Positive people not only have a better chance of avoiding the health problems associated with negative emotions but also tend to have a more efficient immune system. They are also better able to keep their problems in perspective and maintain strong family and social relationships.

The link between our emotions and health is becoming increasingly clear, and it tells us that we can utilize the power of the mind for the benefit of our health. Much research has focused on the ability of the rational mind to influence emotions. The way in which we think and take in, interpret, and remember new information is called cognition. It is this series of cognitive processes that will determine how we feel and respond to a specific situation.

Scientists measure the patterns of cognition by monitoring the different areas of the brain that are active during certain thought processes and by conducting studies into how people solve problems and think their way through situations. The processes that are involved have been shown to be both methodical and complex.

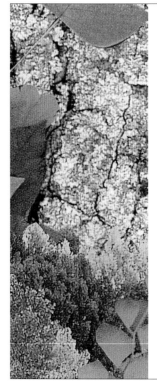

BEING IN CONTROL

One important factor of self-image is how you view events that occur in your life. In the 1950s the psychologist Julian Rotter suggested that people see life in one of two ways: internally or externally. "Internal" people believe that the impetus to shape their lives comes from within each individual, and they enjoy a sense of self-control. "External" persons feel that their lives are out of their personal control, and because of this, they are often inhibited and pressured, seeing themselves as the victims of fate. Predictably, internal per-sons are generally content and happy and are less prone to illness. Look at the chart below

SITUATION	EXTERNAL	INTERNAL
You think that passing an exam depends on	Being lucky with the questions	Preparing thoroughly
You believe that getting a job in which you are happy depends on	Good timing	Working hard to gain the right experience
You think that a successful party depends on	Everybody turning up	Inviting a compatible mix of people
You generally think of yourself as being	Controlled by others	In control of your own destiny
You think that superstitions should be	Observed at all times	Generally laughed at

COGNITIVE THERAPY

In the 1960s Professor Aaron T. Beck pioneered the theory that personal thoughts rather than actual events determine how you feel about something. He claimed that certain types of thinking produce certain types of emotion and that an unrealistic interpretation of an event will skew your emotional response to it.

From this premise he developed cognitive therapy, which aims to correct automatic negative thoughts so that emotional responses become appropriate to the situation. For example, a response such as "this always happens to me" would be questioned by encouraging the person to justify the accuracy of the word *always*. Making the phrase more truthful—saying, for example, "this has happened twice but not at other times, so it isn't inevitable"—helps the person to abandon negative assumptions and learn to see undesired events as temporary setbacks instead of insoluble problems.

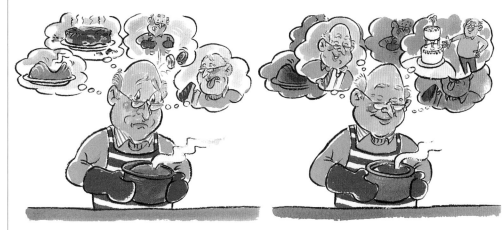

NEGATIVE REINFORCEMENT
It is easy to allow a failure to remind you of other disappointments, reinforcing the impression of failing for most of the time.

THINK POSITIVE
If something goes badly, rather than dwelling on past failures, try to remember the times when things went well.

COGNITIVE PROCESSES

Throughout your life your mind takes in information through the various senses and uses it to build up a mental picture of the world around you. Although this mental picture begins to take shape at a very early age, when you start to distinguish between yourself and the outside world, it is constantly modified as you receive and interpret new information.

Concepts and schemata

Learning to tell the difference between "me" and "not me" is the first step in the formation of concepts and schemata, terms that psychologists use to describe the ways in which you organize and plan your actions.

Concepts help you to construct your picture of the world and to make sense of it by organizing pieces of information into groups that belong together. Your concept of plants, for example, might include trees, flowers, vegetables, and grass, while your concept of animals might include horses, cats, and dogs. One of the most important concepts is that of yourself; it is made up of all the ideas, images, and perceptions that you have as a picture of you.

The term *schema* refers to a more complicated collection of information that includes concepts, memories of past actions or experiences relating to them, and ideas and expectations about possible future actions. You probably have a schema for restaurants, for example, which involves your concept of a restaurant plus your expectations about what will happen when you go into one—for example, being shown to a table and given a menu; ordering, eating, and enjoying your food; and paying for it. So when you go into a restaurant you have

AARON T. BECK
The founder of cognitive therapy, Aaron Beck believed that we have the ability to create our own happiness through careful, positive thinking.

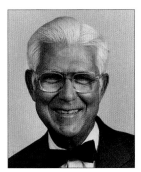

A Woman Fearing Rejection

Anyone who has experienced a traumatic event in childhood will find that its psychological effects persist into adulthood. One common reaction is the belief, either conscious or unconscious, that the event will inevitably repeat itself in some way. This can affect how the person lives and cause difficulties in establishing fulfilling relationships.

Mandy is 34, intelligent, and attractive, and she has a good career and social life. She appears to be the epitome of the successful, confident career woman. In private, however, her life has been a series of painful disappointments. Mandy's parents separated when she was eight, and since that time she has had little contact with her father.

At 24 Mandy fell in love with a man who went off traveling and never returned. Ever since then she has had a series of relationships, none of which have been permanent. After an initial period of romance, she becomes moody and irrational, often provoking fights that end in breakups. Lately she has been suffering persistent headaches and a deepening depression.

WHAT SHOULD MANDY DO?

Mandy must come to terms with her emotional difficulties so that she can start to move forward in her relationships. Underlying her problems is an unconscious conviction that she is unable to sustain loving relationships and that commitment inevitably ends in abandonment. Her lack of self-confidence in this area is affecting her ability to place her trust in a relationship and preventing her from feeling secure or committed.

A therapist might be able to break through this negative thought pattern and help her to focus on the positive aspects of her life. Learning to believe in herself and reconciling to her childhood problems will help change her destructive behavior.

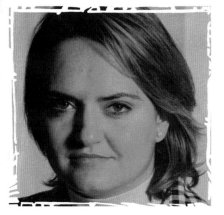

LIFESTYLE
Distorted thinking can lead to negative behavior, which perpetuates emotional problems.

HEALTH
Ill health can often be triggered by negative emotions, which impair the normal functioning of the body and reduce its ability to fight infection.

PARTNERS
Unresolved problems from childhood can carry into adulthood and inhibit the ability to develop healthy relationships.

Action Plan

HEALTH
With the guidance of a therapist, tackle long-term emotional problems. Resolving them can help improve general health.

PARTNERS
Try to approach each new relationship with a sense of freshness. History does not have to repeat itself.

LIFESTYLE
Learn how to recognize and correct the distorted negative thinking that can sabotage personal relationships and lead to depression.

HOW THINGS TURNED OUT FOR MANDY

Mandy went to see a cognitive therapist, who thought that her headaches and moods were linked. He helped her to identify the thought patterns that resulted from her poor self-perception, and together they developed strategies for change. Mandy learned to recognize and check herself when she was slipping into negative thinking. Her headaches have now diminished, and friends have commented that she seems more relaxed.

never visited before, you already have a good idea of what will happen and how you should behave. Without a schema, your visit would be a venture into the unknown. Concepts and schemata enable your mind to make connections quickly between new information and what you already know. In this way you guide your behavior by basing it on previous experiences.

It would be impossible for you to function properly without these mental abilities, but basing your thoughts and actions on prior knowledge and experiences also carries some disadvantages. Significantly, you can develop fixed ways of thinking about certain things that may cloud your judgment and prevent you from adapting to change. Fixed patterns of thinking can make it difficult for you to solve problems because you always opt for tried and tested solutions even when they are not appropriate. They can also influence the way in which you look at and interpret what is happening around you and to you.

Perception is not a straightforward, one-way process in which you simply absorb all the current information about the outside world. Your mind actively selects what information it needs or wants at the time and ignores the rest in order to avoid becoming overloaded and unfocused. It is this selectivity that enables you to concentrate on what one person is saying in a room that is filled with the background chatter of many other people.

This kind of selectivity obviously has its advantages, but difficulties can arise if you are rigidly selective in what you perceive about something or somebody because you have fixed ideas or preconceptions. If you develop a fixed idea about certain people or groups of people—for instance, that they are unlikable or unintelligent—then you will tend to notice their faults more than their good points.

If you develop a fixed idea about yourself, you will probably notice only those things that match your self-perception and disregard any that contradict it. This may not matter much if the fixed idea you have about yourself is relatively positive, but if it is negative, you may end up creating entirely negative thoughts that lead to unhappiness and low self-esteem. These negative

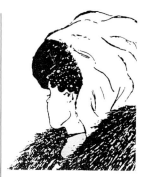

PERCEPTION
The way in which we perceive things can vary dramatically. To some the image above initially appears to be a beautiful young woman, but others first see the face of an old woman.

HOW SCHEMATA WORK

Schemata are cognitive structures that reflect and articulate our knowledge and assumptions about the world. They provide the basic framework for processing information and helping us relate our new experiences to existing knowledge. Once a schema is formed, it will have a strong influence over what we expect and remember from another, similar incident. Our expectations of a restaurant, for example, will have a fixed core—such as expecting to sit at a table and be served—as well as a variable aspect, such as how much the meal will cost or what the food and surroundings will be like.

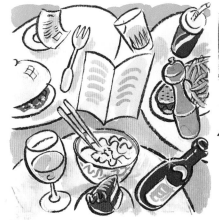

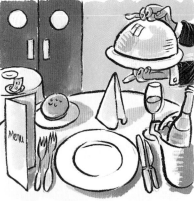

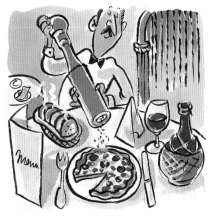

The basic notion of eating out will involve a number of expectations that differ from normal mealtimes. For example, several meal options and a bill for payment will be expected.

An advanced schema for a restaurant will involve more precise ideas about such aspects as service, china, and linens and the way food will be presented.

Further condensation into the schema for a certain type of restaurant, such as an Italian one, will combine the basic expectations with a specific type of food and environment.

THREE STAGES OF MEMORY

Researchers believe that there are three main stages to memory, each differing in capacity, function, and duration. Sensory memory is like a camera, momentarily focusing attention on a detail before taking another shot. The information that you select as important is then transferred to short-term, or working, memory, which holds the material that you are thinking about. Much of the information in this section will be sifted and forgotten until only certain elements are encoded into long-term memory. Information can be stored permanently in long-term memory and recalled into short-term memory when it needs to be thought about. While long-term memory is potentially unlimited, the combination of recollection and new information can cause distortion.

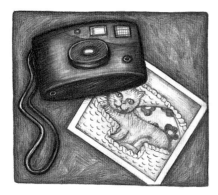

Sensory memory involves split-second images and is informed and constructed by the responses of our senses.

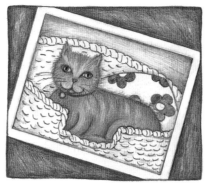

Short-term memory involves the 30 seconds or so spent considering an image or a piece of information.

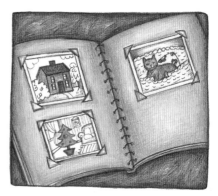

Long-term memory is where we store information. We retrieve and transfer details between this and the short-term memory bank.

emotions, in their turn, tend to reinforce your negative perceptions about both yourself and life in general. Believing that you can never achieve a certain skill or will always embarrass yourself in important social situations, for example, is likely to undermine your confidence further and perpetuate the problem. Seeing yourself as unable to break a cycle of failure will make the act of breaking it far more difficult.

PERCEPTION AND MEMORY

One key contribution to the way we perceive and interpret a situation is our memory. Numerous studies have shown that when we are in a negative mood, we are more likely to recall unhappy memories that will appropriately reinforce our emotions. In a positive frame of mind, we tend to remember happy events that will support our current mood and perpetuate it. Psychologists describe this as mood congruence, and it can significantly alter a person's outlook on life by directing and perpetuating certain emotions. Somebody who tends toward depression, for example, often retrieves memories of personal failure, loss, or pain and subsequently undermines self-confidence even further.

Acknowledging the link between memory and emotion can be useful in directing mood. If you are trying to put yourself into a confident mood, for example, recalling incidences in which you were assertive and strong will help you to feel more powerful. It is easy to let your anxiety take hold, and reminding yourself of times when you were nervous or frightened will only serve to reinforce your fear.

The reliability of memory

We usually believe that if we remember an event in a certain way, then it must, in fact, have been like that. However, our ability to remember things accurately is not clearcut. As we retrieve a memory and reconstruct it in the mind, details can often change, causing errors and distortions that potentially affect our perceptions.

The mind has three stages of memory, and an event needs to be actively processed in each one in order for it to be retained for future use. What we actually store in our long-term memory and the form in which we retrieve it can largely be determined by our schemata. For example, if your schema for relationships is a negative one, you may unconsciously store events that support this attitude and alter details of events so that they fit your schema better. In one experiment conducted by a psychologist in 1980, subjects read a brief story about a happy, compatible couple who were engaged to be married. However, just before leaving, the subjects were told that the couple actually broke up and never did get married. When they were later asked to recall the tale, most people introduced some inaccurate details, such as occasional arguments, in order to make the story consistent with the outcome.

Similarly, eyewitnesses sometimes construct additional information or misidentify criminals because they have distorted events to fit their schema. In 1989 Elizabeth Loftus asked subjects to watch a series of slides in which a burglar used a screwdriver to break into a building. As many as 60 percent of these "witnesses" later claimed to have seen a hammer as one of the intrinsic elements of the crime. The "memories" of these subjects demonstrate how concepts and schemata influence what we remember.

While many cases of forgetfulness and memory distortion are clearly accidental, scientists believe that we may also recall things inaccurately by intention. Just as we may consciously attempt to remember happy memories in a moment of angst, there is evidence to suggest that we may unconsciously suppress negative memories. Some victims of childhood abuse, for example, block out their experiences and are unable to recall any of the details until something happens much later in their lives that triggers the memories.

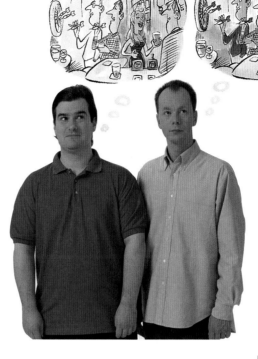

DIFFERENT MEMORIES
Shared experiences can be remembered by people in different ways. One person may recall the presence of a particular person, for example, while another remembers other specific details of the event instead.

POSITIVE AND NEGATIVE THOUGHTS

Sometimes a negative emotion, such as sadness or disappointment, is the appropriate response to an event like the end of a romance or the death of a loved one. At other times, however, negative emotions arise from thoughts that are distorted in some way and are illogical or exaggerated.

These thoughts can be one-time responses to specific events, but they can also be the

CHILD BEHAVIOR

While it is important that parents teach children right and wrong behavior, the manner in which this instruction is delivered can strongly influence self-esteem. Psychologists agree that it is best to try to minimize the pain and discomfort a child feels at moments of disapproval. Strongly expressed anger will have a powerful impact on a young child and can temporarily threaten his or her sense of security within the family unit. Having a good idea of what is expected, acceptable, and consistently approved of provides a child with both the discipline and foundation for good self-esteem in later life. In particular, parents should try to

▶ *call a spade a spade. Labeling behavior as morally wrong when it is simply the result of forgetfulness or procrastination can be confusing. For example, it is inappropriate to call a child "bad" if he or she forgets to tidy a bedroom or is simply putting off the chore.*

▶ *distinguish between criticism of the behavior and criticism of the child. For example, not looking both ways before crossing a road is "bad behavior," not the reflection of a "bad child."*

▶ *be consistent in punishment. If failure to perform chores is greeted with anger on one occasion but shrugged off on the next, the child may become anxious about the apparently arbitrary nature of punishment and confused about the boundaries of right and wrong.*

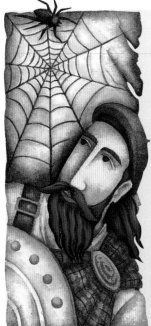

Fables and behavior

ROBERT BRUCE

A classic example of the power of positive thinking is found in the tale of Robert Bruce, who ruled Scotland as Robert I from 1306 to 1329. In 1306, after six failed attempts to rid Scotland of the English king, Edward I, Bruce hid in a cave, feeling despondent. There he watched a spider whose web was damaged six times, and each time it restored the web. Inspired by such determined resilience, Bruce resolved to attempt his coup one more time. Success followed, showing that determination and belief in self can pay off.

result of deep-rooted negative beliefs about the self. Such beliefs can set in at any time in life if self-confidence takes a serious knock. Being bullied or humiliated as a child, for example, or experiencing abandonment or rejection by someone that a person loves can seriously inhibit self-esteem. This in turn leads to distorted thinking in which the individual concentrates on a single negative experience, ignoring all the positive events that should balance it and cancel it out. Like an actor brooding about a negative review and ignoring others that are favorable, some people easily lose sight of the reality of a situation by focusing on certain thoughts and not others.

THE IMPORTANCE OF BUILDING SELF-ESTEEM

Self-esteem is one of the most important contributors to good emotional health. Feeling good about yourself is a vital requirement of personal happiness because it promotes confidence and the belief that you are in control of your life. Conversely, feeling powerless and unhappy with your abilities can affect your attitude and mental capabilities. It is amazing how much personal perception can affect an individual's motivation and behavior. Succeeding in just one difficult task can provide the confidence to take on even greater challenges.

Research suggests that self-esteem has a collective as well as an individual aspect to it. We often evaluate ourselves according to the groups with which we associate, wishing to win our friends' approval and feel at ease within certain social circles. Our self-esteem may be boosted if we perceive that other people view our group favorably, whereas disapproval of our social circle can undermine confidence and lower self-esteem.

The origins of self-esteem

All psychologists agree that much of the groundwork of good self-esteem is laid in childhood. Your parents hug and praise you for behavior they see as appropriate and punish you for dangerous, wrong, or irritating conduct. These memories of approval and disapproval then form the basis of the self-critic within all of us. For this reason it is important to discipline children without undermining their self-esteem.

Most people can remember a case in which a simple comment by a friend or relative stayed with them for several years, affecting their perception and comprehension of the subject and themselves. It is easy to see how an insensitive comment or experience can be taken in the wrong context and undermine a person's self-worth and confidence.

By the time we reach adulthood, we may have taken steps to compensate for areas in which we have failed, in order to restore our sense of self-worth. Clichéd examples of the not very bright child who pursues excellence in sports or the physically weak child who excels academically are demonstrations of how people can learn to compensate for self-perceived failings. Furthermore, as we grow up and mature socially, we become better able to develop friends and relationships on a personal basis. Away from the inescapable grading and limited social choices in childhood, we are able to determine whom we want to have around us; usually they are people who reaffirm our beliefs and outlook. This affirmation often helps provide the self-confidence that many lack, for whatever reason, in the playground.

For all of us, however, self-esteem needs to be reinforced regularly. As adults, we still encounter situations that can undermine our confidence, and while we may be better at handling such situations, it's important to acknowledge our emotions and reaffirm our self-esteem. Sometimes therapy or counseling are necessary to deal with low self-esteem, but there is also much we can do to help strengthen it ourselves.

CHALLENGING YOUR THOUGHT PATTERNS

There is much you can do to change negative ways of thinking. Visualization exercises and relaxation therapies can be of particular benefit in promoting positive thought.

Changing your way of thinking for the better is always possible, even if the thought patterns you wish to change are long-standing and ingrained. First you need to examine your ideas and beliefs to find out whether or not they are valid. Then you can start to shed or revise those that aren't helpful and create new ones that are. This exercise will provide you with a more positive belief system and give you the ability to recognize and prevent other negative, self-destructive thoughts. Should you have any doubt about your ability to change your thoughts and beliefs, just look back over your life and consider all of the revisions you have already made. Making the transition from childhood to adulthood, establishing relationships, leaving your childhood home, and finding one or more jobs—all involve making decisions and adaptations in your lifestyle. While many of these decisions may have been forced on you by circumstances,

ENCOURAGING OPENNESS

Having confidence in your thoughts and beliefs allows you to be your most natural self. Understanding how and why you think as you do can help you to have more confidence in your own capabilities. The following visualization is particularly good for encouraging openness in your attitude toward others and in helping you accept and appreciate your own individual characteristics.

Sit or lie down in a quiet place.

Imagine your heart opening up and encompassing all of you.

Inside are all the good and bad bits, the qualities that you like about yourself and the characteristics that you don't. As your heart embraces you in your entirety, understand that it loves all of you. You are yourself and that is sufficient.

Now imagine this love extending into the room and beyond your house, to all the people you know.

Invite these people to join you and share in the self-love that is overflowing from your heart. Picture yourself playing with the others, enjoying independence, confidence, and individuality. Accept the idea that you will always have the freedom to simply be yourself.

COGNITIVE DISSONANCE

Most people at some time will experience difficulty in maintaining harmony between their actions and their beliefs. The anxiety we feel in observing the inconsistencies between our thoughts and actions is known as cognitive dissonance. Psychologists believe that we learn to reconcile these difficulties in one of three key ways. A smoker aware of the harmful effects of nicotine, for example, may resort to one of the following behaviors:

▶ *Action and belief are reconciled as the person accepts the dangers of smoking and subsequently gives up the habit.*

▶ *The belief is counteracted with arguments that seem to disprove it, such as examples of a smoker who lived a long time and did not suffer any health problems.*

▶ *The issue is played down so that the dissonance no longer seems important. Arguing that we must die from something and that it may as well be through pleasure is a common example.*

they still show that it is possible to revise and alter your beliefs when the situation calls for doing so.

CHALLENGING YOUR OWN IDEAS

It is not practical or perhaps even feasible to try to change all of your incorrect ideas, assumptions, and beliefs in one try. The best approach is to deal with them one by one when they arise. When something troubles you, making you unhappy, anxious, or stressed, use the opportunity to examine the ideas and beliefs that underpin your reaction. If you catch yourself thinking a negative thought, challenge its validity by examining the evidence and support for your reaction. For example, if you think that everything you do is never good enough, ask yourself why you believe improvement to be impossible. Similarly, ask yourself whether others would agree with your judgment.

Many people are too hard on themselves, mentally berating themselves for an action that would not even warrant mild criticism from a friend, spouse, or colleague. Indeed, if another person made the same mistake, you would probably offer understanding and support, perhaps giving only gentle and constructive criticism. Treating yourself as compassionately as you treat others can go a long way toward maintaining mental well-being. If you do have a negative thought, question its benefits. If it has any at all, compare them with the mental advantages of dismissing the thought and replacing it with a positive one. Negative thoughts seldom have much to offer, and their principal effect is generally to breed further negativity.

OVERCOMING NEGATIVITY

An excellent visualization for overcoming negative thoughts involves realizing and accepting how many expectations we put on ourselves. As adults, we attempt increasingly to suppress or hide our failings, trying to be perfect and suffering personal retribution for mistakes. Imagining yourself as a child with no pressure to maintain a certain image can help to reduce intense self-criticism.

Visualize your inner self, perhaps as an innocent child who still feels free to act and behave without inhibition. Try to remember how it felt to simply be yourself.

Sit or lie somewhere comfortable and peaceful.

Now talk to your inner child. Apologize for leaving it behind and trying to deny its natural instincts and fallibility. Promise to be more open to it.

IMPROVING YOUR SELF-ESTEEM

To improve your self-esteem, you need to take a positive view of yourself and your abilities. A good first step in recognizing your positive qualities is to make them the focus of your self-perception. Drawing up a list of your good points and reading them whenever you feel down will help to remind you of your own strengths and abilities.

The second step is to make a list of your faults and look at them objectively, considering whether any of them can be seen in a more positive light. For instance, if one item on your list is "I tend to be rude to other people," you could see this as "I'm honest with people about how I feel." Then try to accentuate the positive aspect and reduce the negative aspect—saying, for example, "I will be honest with people, but I will try to be tactful." Following through on these intentions and making an effort to fulfill them is a positive act that will in itself help to raise your self-esteem.

Question your "shoulds"

Your "shoulds" are those beliefs and values acquired at an early age that tell you how to behave and what you should say and do. Most of these are perfectly reasonable, but any that aren't will make demands on you that may be difficult to meet. An excessive tendency toward guilt, for example, can make you feel unworthy when you're not, while a belief that you should never make mistakes will set up a pattern of unrealistic expectations and subsequent dismay.

Making choices

No matter how strong and resilient you try to make your self-esteem, there will inevitably be occasions when things go wrong. In these instances it is important not to fall into the trap of believing that this failure indicates a general character defect. By treating each event as a one-time occurrence and attempting to learn from the experience, you can feel more confident about doing better in the future.

The personal intensity of a failure can help to determine how much it will affect your self-esteem. While a whole host of minor failings may leave you fairly unperturbed, one single failure involving a deeply held belief may be completely devastating. Similarly, a single success or affirmation of approval has the potential to reinforce your self-esteem far more than a series of minor accomplishments.

Imagine yourself in a world where your inner child is completely free. Picture the child running and playing, making mistakes but remaining happy and confident.

Now picture yourself in the same world. Combine with your inner child so that you are connected and experience the same things. This will help you to release future emotions more readily.

Ultimately, these conflicts of interest occur because we have to make choices involving priorities. Choosing whom we wish to please most—our parents, partner, boss, or self, for instance—will affect how we maintain and boost self-esteem. While it would be nice to please everybody all the time, reality dictates that this is not possible. Learning to expect but not fear occasional shortcomings will help strengthen your self-esteem.

YOUR THOUGHT POLICE

Once you become aware of your negative thoughts and beliefs, it should be relatively easy to recognize any new ones that arise. Quickly dismissing or replacing these thoughts before they multiply or take hold is particularly important for maintaining mental balance. Do not let one incident lead to a negative train of thinking.

Try to avoid continual worrying as well. While anxiety is often justifiable as a response to particular situations, all-pervasive, perpetual worrying can be harmful to both your physical health and your peace of mind. Focus your attention on the real scale of any problem and constructively work through your options. This will help to divert your thoughts away from the event and toward some action.

SELF-SUFFICIENCY

The term *self-sufficiency* refers to an individual's expectations and belief in his or her capabilities. Having the confidence to try to control events in your life can have a major effect on your behavior and boost your ability to withstand stress. An effective way to build up your self-sufficiency is to take proper notice of your successes. By concentrating on the positive side of your abilities, you will become more confident in coping with future situations that are stressful.

While you should approach challenges with vigor, it's also important to set realistic aims because too much ambition can lead to failure and disillusionment. Such failures may then undermine the very confidence on which you rely. Setting realistic incentives and perhaps offering yourself appropriate rewards may help to inspire you for future achievements and reinforce your confidence.

DEAL WITH YOUR INTERNAL CRITIC
Your internal critic is the voice in your head that puts you down every time you fail or make a mistake. Talking back to your critic and identifying any half truths can help you to achieve a more realistic evaluation of yourself.

DID YOU KNOW?
Most people reaffirm their beliefs unconsciously. We not only buy newspapers and magazines that reflect our point of view but also read articles in a certain way. We tend to dismiss points with which we disagree and focus on arguments that reinforce and confirm our own beliefs.

Relearning anticipation

One common complaint about growing older is that things no longer seem so exciting. We inhibit or lose a sense of anticipation and no longer get as much pleasure from favorite activities or good friends as we used to. Believing that holidays or birthdays are not as good as they used to be, however, commonly leads us to feel less enthusiastic about such events and inevitably to gain less enjoyment from them.

Although a diminished sense of anticipation can affect the ultimate pleasure derived from an event, it is still possible for the event to be rewarding. Dreading the prospect of a dinner party but enjoying it when you are there is a common example of why negative anticipation should not be allowed to dictate your actual response.

Try this exercise to help you relearn anticipation. Choose four or five activities that you expect to complete this week. These targets should be ordinary occurrences, such as gardening or having lunch with a friend. After writing down each event, note three reasons why you will enjoy it. Simple acts like choosing plants or catching up on gossip, for example, help to make an event pleasurable. Analyzing what makes something appealing when you are experiencing it can help you to relearn a sense of anticipation and look forward to an event.

Positive life events

One of the best ways to help yourself cope with everyday problems and pressures is to make a point of regularly counterbalancing them with pleasures. Setting aside a little time each day to relax and do something that you enjoy will prevent niggling problems from dominating your life. Holidays, hobbies, and sports are physically and mentally beneficial as well as enjoyable. They can give you the foundation to believe in your own power and abilities.

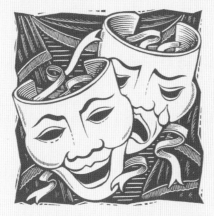

CHAPTER 4

LEARNING ABOUT EMOTIONS

A normal, healthy person experiences a whole range of emotions, both good and bad, that manifest themselves mentally and physically. But dealing with feelings, especially those we like least, and assessing how appropriate a response is can be difficult. This chapter examines the different emotions that everybody experiences from time to time and looks at how to channel them constructively.

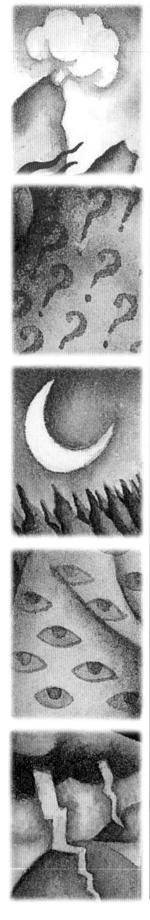

EXAMINING EMOTIONS

We all experience love, anger, sadness, and joy but perhaps are less aware of the vast range of intensity that each of these emotions encompasses.

All of the emotions that people feel, including happiness, sadness, love, anxiety, fear, loneliness, and anger, are necessary aspects of good health. They demonstrate that we are sufficiently receptive to our environment to be affected by it. We are biologically programmed to have and express feelings and are socially encouraged to share these emotions because of a common cultural need.

When the intensity of feelings becomes excessive, however, the results can be problematic. We can all remember incidences in which anger got the better of us and was disproportionate to the situation or when love perhaps blinded our judgment. While it is perfectly normal to feel occasionally overcome with emotion, most people would agree that frequent excessive responses can be physically and mentally damaging. For example, sadness and grief express inner turmoil and can be a good way of working through pain before moving on. But if these sources of inspiration are allowed to gain a negative hold and take control of your life, the result can be depression. It is important to find a balance between expressing your emotions and appropriately controlling them, but the effort can be difficult.

External influences

The ability to express a mood or feeling varies greatly among individuals. It is in part determined by attitudes developed in childhood and depends on whether or not children are encouraged to be emotionally open and honest. In some cultures—Mediterranean, for instance—people are inherently expressive about their feelings, whereas in others—Anglo-Saxon, for example—they tend to repress or deny some of their natural feelings because the society deems it appropriate. No matter what the culture has dictated, however, women have been stereotypically associated with more emotional behavior than men for much of the history of Western civilization. Now the idea has taken hold that men have just as much need and right to express their feelings as women do.

Of course, these are generalizations, and no two individuals will ever feel or act in exactly the same way, but a person's emotional openness tends to depend on personal and social expectations rather than biological tendencies. While all people experience grief, for instance, some cultures encourage open expression of the feeling, and others expect suppression of it. Essentially, our emotional honesty is determined by many factors, including cultural, social, and personal expectations and attitudes.

Some common perceptions

There are many different theories about what constitutes good emotional health, but the common thread seems ultimately to be about balance. Most therapists believe in a natural inner harmony that can be restored through self-awareness. This means using and relieving your feelings constructively and aiming to return ultimately to a happy, balanced state. Eastern philosophies have always asserted the importance of energy fields in influencing mood and behavior, and now Western attitudes are increasingly coming around to the idea of a relationship between physical and mental balance. Philosophies from Ayurveda to Taoism to Zen all assert that we can counteract excessive emotions and maintain or return to a state of balanced wholeness.

THE FIVE ENERGIES

While we might all be vaguely familiar with a certain feeling of optimism in spring or lethargy in autumn, Chinese philosophy asserts that different times of the year can and do have very definite effects on our moods. The natural change in energy levels with each shift of the weather can affect our temperament, causing imbalances that can distort or determine mood. This concept is similar to the theory of seasonal affective disorder (see page 101). According to Chinese philosophy, everything moves in one continual energy flow and this flow needs to be balanced in order to keep your life on course. Spring to midsummer is associated with the vital energies of yang, while the quieter qualities of yin become dominant toward autumn, bringing with them a different set of emotional tendencies.

The five seasons of Chinese philosophy—spring, summer, late summer, autumn, and winter—are paralleled by five elements that reflect the energy forces to be balanced. The young, expansive qualities of wood symbolize the youthful vitality of spring, incorporating the human tendency to be passionate in such emotions as anger and love. In the yin season of winter, the element of water takes precedence as coldness leads to states of tension and apprehension. In the yang vibrancy of early summer, however, the creative power of fire warms the blood and causes people to experience intense sensations of joy or hate.

Just as each element relates to a season and type of emotion, it is also believed to relate to a particular organ, demonstrating how the body, the mind, and the physical environment are all interconnected in one driving force. The winter element of water, for example, is associated with the kidneys and bladder, whereas fiery summer, with its intense passions of hate or joy, is identified with the heart. Physical problems with circulation or excessively passionate feelings of hate, for example, will be seen as symptomatic of too much yang energy in the summer element. To restore balance among the patient's physical organs, emotional state, and general sense of well-being, a traditional Chinese doctor might prescribe calming yin type foods, such as blackberries, watermelon, or pears, for this condition.

FIVE ELEMENTS THEORY
Chinese medicine uses the concept of five elements in the diagnosis and treatment of physical and emotional imbalances. Each element has its own correlations with organs, mood states, a color, and a season.

Fire
The red of fire is related to early summer and the intense passions of hate and joy. Physically, it is linked to the heart and circulatory system.

Earth
In addition to the four seasons of Western tradition, the Chinese include a fifth—late summer. Its predominant color is yellow, and it is associated with feelings of empathy and organs near the stomach, such as the pancreas.

Wood
The youthful strength of wood represents vitality and the green of spring. Associated with the liver and the gallbladder, it symbolizes the emotions of anger and kindness.

Water
Representing the coolness of winter, water affects the kidneys and bladder and is represented by the color black. It symbolizes the qualities of spontaneity, fear, and calmness.

Metal
The element of autumn, metal is associated with the colon and lungs. It is represented by the color white and the sensations of grief and courage.

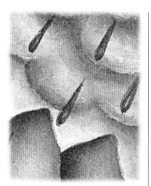

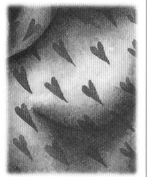

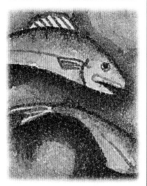

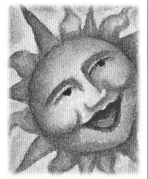

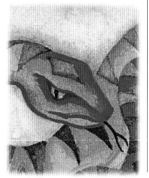

AYURVEDA

Ayurveda is an ancient Indian medical practice and philosophy with many concepts similar to those of Chinese medicine. Ayurveda seeks to balance the body and the mind by combining five elements—water, fire, earth, air, and ether—in a healthy balance. Three bioenergies, or *tridoshas,* are divided into *vata,* a combination of ether and air, *pitta,* composed of fire with a little water, and *kapha,* a combination of water and earth. In an ideal state, all three doshas should be in perfect balance, but according to Ayurvedic principle, most of us have an imbalance that makes us more inclined toward one or perhaps two of these states. The dosha that dominates the body also gives rise to a certain physical and emotional type.

If you are primarily vata, you are likely to be quick and imaginative, a changeable person who is always on the go and prone to anxiety. Those of a pitta disposition are usually quite determined and courageous, good organizers who tend to react angrily when things go wrong. Kapha people are generally calm; they crave security and prefer easygoing, regulated lifestyles with slow, methodical activities.

Finding your type

Ayurvedic theory accepts that we all behave differently but asserts that we lean toward one or other of the dosha types, and it is by balancing out our excesses that we can achieve true emotional health.

Keeping yourself in balance involves first recognizing when you are displaying excessive characteristics of a particular dosha. A vata person may easily become overanxious, for example, or a pitta person may become excessively irritable. These characteristics can then be adjusted by taming your lifestyle, eating certain foods, or doing an appropriate exercise to restore harmony. For example, a person with excessive vata tendencies should avoid too many stimulants, such as loud noise or action, whereas people who are predominantly kapha might seek a little more excitement in their lives in order to prevent lethargy.

The basic principle is to recognize and accept your prevailing dosha type and keep it in balance with the less predominant ones. This will help you feel better both physically and mentally, improving fitness, concentration, and the ability to relax.

BACH FLOWER REMEDIES

Although the Bach Flower remedies were developed in the West, the theory behind them shares some of the concepts of Eastern philosophies. Dr. Edward Bach, a British physician, believed that the whole patient should be treated—not his disease. Instead of just prescribing drugs to treat symptoms of illness, a medical practitioner should consider a patient's personality and state of mind in deciding on a course of treatment.

Bach also believed that negative mental states and emotional imbalances are at the root of inner conflicts and tensions and are the ultimate cause of ill health and unhappiness. He studied the plants in the countryside of England and Wales and developed 38 natural plant remedies to relieve specific negative emotions and imbalances and thus enable patients to establish a foundation for good physical and mental health. He also created a combination formula—the rescue remedy—which is meant to be used as an emergency treatment in moments of crisis.

The remedies are prepared today using the same methods that Bach devised. Flowers are immersed in spring water and left in the sun for three hours or parts of plants are boiled in spring water for half an hour. The plants are then discarded and the water is preserved in brandy as a tincture.

Emotional variation

Nobody knows exactly how Bach remedies work, but they are completely natural and cause no ill side effects. A significant aspect of successful use of the remedies lies in accurately determining the psychological state underlying a particular emotion. This self-analysis can in itself have a therapeutic effect.

Some emotions have one particular flower associated with them, whereas others have several, reflecting how the same emotion may be caused by different mental states. Similarly, two different remedies may be identified with a particular emotion, but one may help deal with an excess of it and the other with a deficiency. For example, some people may wish to overcome their feelings of loneliness, while others may feel that they crave solitude too much and need a remedy to restore emotional equilibrium.

The chart on the opposite page identifies a selection of key emotions and their variations, alongside Bach's suggested remedy for each case.

BACH FLOWER REMEDIES

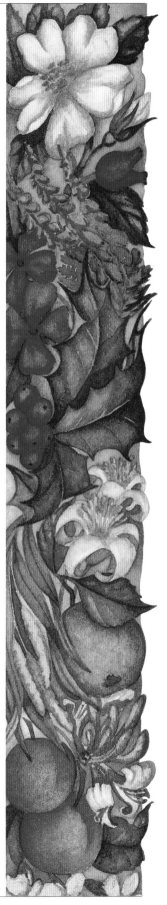

EMOTION OR STATE OF MIND	DESCRIPTION	FLOWER
Ambition	Overly ambitious Lacking in ambition	Rock water; vervain Clematis; wild rose
Anger	Easily angered; intolerant Feeling out of control; impulsive	Beech Cherry plum
Assertiveness (lack of)	Easily exploited Lacking in confidence	Centaury Larch
Anxiety or apprehension	Fearing everyday things; phobic	Aspen; mimulus
Broodiness	Tendency to dwell on the past	Honeysuckle
Concern (excessive)	About others; possessive For own welfare For minor issues; feeling shame	Chicory; red chestnut Heather; rock water Crab apple
Conflict (fear of)	Finding arguments distressing	Agrimony; centaury
Depression	Resulting from small setbacks Resulting from feelings of inferiority For no apparent reason	Gentian Larch Holly; mustard
Despondency	Feeling despair or gloom	Sweet chestnut; mustard
Discouragement	Feeling overwhelmed; self-pitying	Elm; willow
Domineering	Demanding much of others	Vine
Fear	Of rejection Of failure Of losing control Of threatening situations	Centaury; larch Mimulus Aspen Rock rose
Guilt	Tendency to blame self Tendency to blame others	Pine Willow
Hate	Quickly arising hatred	Holly; willow
Indecision	Difficulty in making decisions quickly	Cerato; scleranthus
Inhibition	Shy with others; unapproachable	Larch; water violet
Instability	Feeling shaky and out of balance	Scleranthus
Jealousy and envy	Needing more love; resentful	Holly; willow
Loneliness	Do not want to be alone Prefer to be alone	Chicory; heather Clematis; impatiens
Melancholy	Tendency to pessimism or gloom	Gentian; mustard
Need to adapt	Experiencing transition or new beginning	Walnut
Obsessive	Experiencing recurring unwanted thoughts	White chestnut
Overenthusiastic	Needing to convince or convert others	Vervain
Stressed	Putting excessive pressure on self	Elm; rock water
Stuck in a rut	Finding no joy; drifting through life	Wild rose

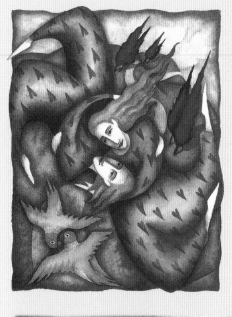

Love

Love, a difficult concept to define, means something different to everybody. From the compassionate love of friendship to the passionate experiences of romance to the love between parent and child, we each have our own expectations of this emotion.

Different kinds of love

Our first experiences of love come from the early relationships we develop with family and friends. While our role as a son or daughter does not involve intense sensations of passion, the qualities of respect, commitment, support, and compassion are all set up in these initial stages. When our parents provide nurturing guidance, we learn to trust, developing our independence while still being enfolded in and relying on the support of a secure, loving unit. The foundation of such love lies in the biology of survival, the need to be cared for, nurtured, and provided with the confidence and self-esteem to face the outside world.

The inherent desire and need for love and support that we develop in these early stages set up the basis for our future lives. Constantly seeking and maintaining friendships, we realize the importance of a supportive unit that offers similar levels of compassion and commitment. Many close, platonic friendships can embody the same levels of respect, tolerance, and loyalty, the same importance to daily life, as more intimate associations can. Nevertheless, in addition to many loving platonic connections, most people also wish to enjoy the intimacy of a sexual relationship.

Although we all exist as independent individuals, external factors contribute to a general sense of needing one-to-one intimacy and affection. While biology dictates that we should reproduce in order to aid the survival of the species, cultural influences suggest that it is normal to seek out and settle down with a partner with whom you feel comfortable. Modern Western society, with its increased emphasis on independence and greater acceptance of homosexuality, has somewhat altered the traditional view, but it seems that regardless of sexual orientation, age, or lifestyle, we are still expected to be searching for love. Part of the reason for this is that love in modern society does not have to serve a specific function. Many people claim that the person on whom they have settled does not conform to any of the expectations or ideals with which they set out. Instead, love often happens against their better judgment, causing intense feelings of passion, adoration, and respect. It is partly a natural instinct to love and be loved, a way of reaffirming one's self-esteem.

Many theories have tried to explain why we fall in love with a particular person. While some people believe that opposites attract, others argue that we gravitate toward someone who shares much in common with us. Most people, however, probably fall somewhere in the middle, seeking a person with some characteristics similar to their own while still accepting some interesting differences. Many people fall in love with someone who presents the same challenges as those experienced in early childhood, suggesting that we seek comfort in the familiar or are perhaps trying to resolve "unfinished business." Women with distant fathers, for example, may tend to fall in love with emotionally distant men, while some men yearn for a maternal figure. We all have our own foibles and attractions, many of which, just like love itself, cannot be logically rationalized.

> *"When Love speaks, the voice of all the gods makes heaven drowsy with the harmony."*

WILLIAM SHAKESPEARE

Falling in love

The difficulty of defining or explaining the attraction of one person to another lies partly in different aspirations. The kind of relationship that each person seeks can vary. While some individuals crave spontaneous, unqualified passion, others look for the companionable love that can sustain a long-term marriage or partnership. Most people, however, would agree that they feel little rational judgment when choosing a potential mate. Falling in love can be both illogical and inconvenient, disrupting an individual's life and perception and forcing him or her to find compromises between expectations and reality. Indeed, few people rationally choose the individuals with whom they fall in love. Nevertheless, the magical intensity of falling in love can be thrilling. The immediate sensations of an all-encompassing world, the flattery of having your feelings reciprocated, and the romance of enjoying a new set of experiences encourage us to seek out this emotion.

Yet it is inevitable that as time passes, the shortcomings and weaknesses of each partner start to show and the thrill can begin to wear off. Such disillusionment is perhaps the greatest test of true love. Most successful long-term relationships rely on both partners accepting constructive change. In order to be sustained, love must inevitably mature, and commitment, tolerance, and emotional intimacy are far more likely to sustain a loving relationship than overwhelming sexual passion or unrealistic expectations. The true nature of lasting love usually involves having the emotional maturity to deal with these changes.

Obsession and possessiveness

Obsession is a form of anxiety in which persistent, repetitive thoughts, feelings, or ideas take over a person's consciousness. In extreme cases the person may feel possessed by the obsession, sometimes in spite of being aware of its destructiveness and even while wishing it would stop.

Being obsessed about someone you love or being the object of someone's obsession may seem romantic, but it makes developing a realistic relationship impossible. If you are obsessed, you may idealize the person, projecting onto him or her everything you hope to find in a partner, whether or not such attributes really exist. That same person, if assessed objectively, may feel threatened by such intensity of feeling or behavior.

Jealous possessiveness of another person tends to preclude the possibility of developing a genuinely healthy relationship. Some parents are possessive of their children, which can inhibit the children's ability to grow up and cause their resentment and eventual alienation. And some people find it difficult to accept the independence and individuality of their partners. In many of these cases, lack of self-confidence and self-esteem often lies at the root of the problem.

A person who fears rejection or loneliness may be unable to enter into a relationship with adult maturity and will resort to negative behavior in order to reinforce self-esteem.

Despite the attraction of an intimate relationship, it is important not to let the desire for love obscure your perspective. The loyalty and compassion of friends and family may not provide passionate fervor, but they can do much to reinforce your sense of self-worth.

BRINGING MORE LOVE INTO YOUR LIFE

If you generally have difficulty in forming loving relationships, it may help to examine your self-perception. Perhaps you have an underlying belief that you are unable to sustain a relationship, and this belief could be affecting the way in which you approach intimate friendships. Concentrating on yourself may sound selfish, but it is a good way to build a foundation for loving intimacy. Learning to trust and like yourself should help to make you more receptive to and able to sustain healthy, loving relationships. Consider some of the following points.

- *Not having an intimate relationship does not mean that you are unloved if you have the support of your friends and family; this will be there at all times—even during the rocky moments of a partnership.*

- *Obsessively seeking love can actually be counterproductive because overwhelming neediness repels potential friends and partners. By diverting your attention to new hobbies and other activities, you can refocus your self-consciousness and at the same time make a greater number of new friends and acquaintances.*

- *Focusing on the positive aspects of your life is reaffirming. Friendships, good family relationships, career success, and absorbing hobbies all demonstrate the many successes in your life and your ability to be self-sufficient.*

- *Most people spend a substantial amount of time being single and content before entering the complicated world of relationship seeking. This shows that it is possible to be happy and fulfilled without intimate love. Each stage of life offers different opportunities.*

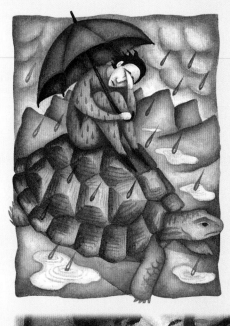

Sadness and grief

Everyone experiences sadness and grief at some point in their lives. Major events such as bereavement, divorce, or losing a job, or even lesser disappointments like the defeat of a favorite team, can cause pain and sorrow as an individual is forced to come to terms with an unwanted situation or outcome.

The difference between sadness and grief

There is a distinction between sadness and grief. Sadness tends to be associated with a sense of unhappiness, sorrow, or regret. This feeling may result from a particular disappointment, such as the cancellation of a long-awaited event, or may arise from a more general sense of unhappiness or disappointment, for example, over the direction that a person's life seems to be taking. Grief, on the other hand, follows a highly distressing experience that is usually related to another person, such as a death, separation, or divorce. In these circumstances sorrow may be accompanied by other, more complex emotions—disbelief, numbness, shock, denial, yearning, pining, despair, or depression, for example. All or some of these feelings may be experienced in different degrees and combinations.

Another important difference between sadness and grief is that sadness is usually experienced as a temporary state of mind, lasting just hours or days. Grief,

however, is usually experienced for several months and can even last for years, depending on the closeness of the relationship with the other person.

The complex sensations of loss and despair can be bound up with other conflicting emotions, such as anger that a loved one has gone. Many people often feel a sense of relief too, particularly if the departed person was suffering from severe pain for a long time before dying. This emotion can in turn trigger other reactions, such as a sense of confusion or guilt at feeling relieved.

Although grief is usually thought of in relation to the loss of or separation from a loved person, the need to mourn can be a natural response to other major events involving loss. These might include the loss of a pet with whom a person has developed deep emotional ties or being laid off after many years in a job. Parents may even feel grief when their children leave home, experiencing the so-called empty nest syndrome.

The grieving process often follows a distinct sequence, starting with shock and protest and passing through despair and denial before culminating in a sense of detachment. However, a bereaved person may remain in one stage of grief and find it difficult to move on. A widower stuck in denial, for example, may eventually suffer delusions, refusing to accept that his wife's death actually occurred. Or a grieving widow may continue to refer to her husband in the present tense, listen for his key in the door, and even cook him a meal.

Being angry at the loved one for dying, weeping uncontrollably, holding imaginary conversations with the deceased, having hallucinations of seeing the dead person, and dreaming that he or she is still alive are all common reactions. Grieving people may also unconsciously mimic a beloved dead person's behavior or speech patterns.

However painful it may be, the process of grieving is not an illness but an inevitable life experience that offers potential for growth. Widows who previously relied entirely on their husbands in practical and financial matters, for example, have the opportunity to grow into self-sufficiency. And many people find a new or renewed sense of spirituality.

"Give sorrow words: the grief that does not speak
Whispers the o'er-fraught heart and bids it break."

WILLIAM SHAKESPEARE

78

Depression and melancholia

The sadness associated with bereavement is a normal part of grieving but can often lead to depression. Sigmund Freud called this emotional state melancholia. Symptoms of depression include dejection and hopelessness, lack of self-esteem, loss of interest in life, and an inability to give or receive love or lead a normal, active life.

Depression may occur only intermittently during the initial period of grieving—at the funeral, for example, or when divorce papers are finalized—as earlier defense mechanisms, such as denial, break down. When the reality and finality of the loss can no longer be avoided, depression can become pervasive and life may seem meaningless.

At this stage a bereaved person may be perfectly able to carry out day-to-day tasks with little apparent show of emotion. This is often taken by others to indicate that the grieving person is getting over the loss when, in fact, his or her depression may continue privately for months to come. This is especially true of children, who often seem to recover rapidly from the loss of a parent or sibling while actually remaining depressed.

Severe, prolonged depression is the most common form of mental illness associated with grief. Contributing factors include a genetic predisposition to depression, the death of a parent, and irrational delusions of guilt and self-blame. (Chapter 5 explores these issues in greater depth.)

Loneliness, isolation, and highly ambivalent or negative feelings about the lost one can intensify depression. The loss of a spouse whose profession gave the bereaved person a well-defined identity—a clergyman or diplomat, for example—can also increase these depressive feelings.

Coping with grief

Coming to terms with grief can be very difficult, and the subsequent emotional turmoil is often especially trying. Constantly reminding yourself that things will get better is often the only way to pull yourself through this period. Both grief and loss are subjective experiences, and no one but you can fully understand your emotional anguish.

Although most people share similar reactions to particular events, the intensity of these experiences and their means of expression are always highly individual. There is never one correct way to grieve or express sorrow, and personal reactions will vary.

While some people break down with little provocation, others find it extremely hard to release their grief. This inability can lead to a dangerous accumulation of emotion. Many people are surprised by the apparent irrationality of their feelings, finding it difficult to grieve openly for the loss of a loved one, yet weeping quite freely at the news of being laid off from work.

Remember that seeking and accepting help is an act of strength rather than weakness. Working through your grief will help you come to terms with your feelings and emerge in a more positive frame of mind rather than with a suppressed or overwhelming burden. By experiencing your grief, you gradually process it, and this allows you to resume a normal life. Feeling guilty about your thoughts, behavior, or feelings or trying to deny or repress grief is counterproductive. The grief simply lies hidden, only to return with the next loss, perhaps causing unbearable feelings.

A family doctor may initially prescribe a mild tranquilizer, but emotional support and a willingness to listen are often more important. A strong support network of family and friends also helps.

RELEASING GRIEF AND SADNESS

Both sadness and grief need to be expressed in an individual, subjective way to be of any emotional benefit. Acknowledging your emotion is the best way to relieve it, although you must find a way to release it that will work well for you.

■ *Many people find that the simple act of crying is the best way of releasing emotional pain.*

■ *Maintaining a busy and fulfilling routine, as long as you don't use work to hide from your feelings, is a good way to prevent yourself from dwelling on problems.*

■ *Taking a rest whenever you feel either physically or emotionally drained is helpful.*

■ *Remember that overwhelming sensations of sorrow and grief do lessen with time. Meanwhile, try to express your feelings and share your pain with your partner, friends, or relatives. Your doctor can also provide support and, if necessary, medication.*

■ *While you should avoid living in the past, it is also important to avoid going to the other extreme and making too many life-changing decisions at this time. Remember that you are now in a period of transition, and making a dramatic change in terms of career or lifestyle at this point will intensify rather than relieve any feelings of insecurity that you might have.*

■ *Consider getting counseling or psychotherapy, which has helped many people to cope during times of heightened sorrow or bereavement. In this case the professional's role is often to provide a focus for the feelings of pent-up anger and frustration that cannot be directed at anyone else.*

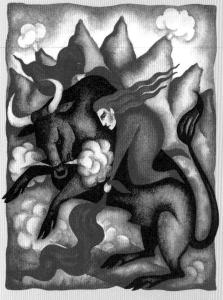

Anger

Anger is an extreme and passionate emotion that has considerable physiological effects. It can be brought on by any number of different experiences and may present problems both in terms of its expression and its suppression.

Learning from anger and aggression

Anger is among the earliest feelings experienced by an infant and is one of the most important emotions a person possesses. In most instances anger serves as a basic survival mechanism; when we feel threatened in any way, the anger response prepares the body for physical action—"fight or flight." While anger can be a problematic emotion for some people, understanding that it is, at heart, a self-preservation mechanism, often based on fear, can help you to deal constructively with its effects.

Anger and aggression are common and sometimes necessary, but the way in which an individual manages and expresses them will determine how constructive they are. Used carefully and in a controlled way, anger and even occasional aggression can be effective in achieving a desired result. Shouting at a child who runs out into a busy road without looking, for example, should provide enough of a shock effect to prevent a similar occurrence. Unbridled anger or aggression, however, is almost invariably counterproductive. While your

reasons for being angry may be perfectly valid, having continuous outbursts or resorting to physical violence will set up an ineffective communication pattern. The recipient will respond with his or her own defense mechanisms, such as defiance, aggression, or withdrawal, thus reducing the likelihood of effective communication. Continuous parental outbursts of anger, for example, will eventually lose their effectiveness as a source of discipline or appropriate emotion. The child will no longer equate specific naughty actions with anger and will lose respect for the emotion.

An adult who responds angrily most of the time may also find that other people avoid interaction of any kind. The social implications of unrelenting anger are at best mild irritation, at worst complete social breakdown. Fortunately, very few people take anger to the extremes of road-rage attacks and physical violence. Nonetheless, low-level but constant anger or aggression invariably causes the recipient to at least avoid, if not actively shun, the aggressor.

If anger seems grossly exaggerated in relation to the alleged cause, it may be fueled by some unresolved issues. Repeated and unjustified punishment during childhood, for example, may lead to enormous fury at a mild accusation in adulthood. Or an outburst at one incident may actually be relief from other, more pressing situations.

Some outbursts have no apparent cause, apart from accumulated frustration. People who allow situations and feelings to build up and avoid addressing a problem often set up emotional stress that must ultimately be released in anger.

All emotions need to be articulated in order to relieve the tension that they engender; a simple blush, for example, is the body's physiological release from feelings of embarrassment or shyness. Denying or suppressing a natural reaction like anger can be self-destructive. Turned in on itself, anger can build up to a dangerous point, eventually being expressed in a sudden, violent outburst or through chronic physical symptoms, such as stress and depression. It is very important therefore to understand the physiological effects of anger and to find ways of releasing your anger that will limit the destructive elements of the emotion and channel its positive force.

"Anger is one of the sinews of the soul."

THOMAS FULLER

80

Physical effects of anger

There is evidence that continuously high levels of anger pose a serious threat to health. Research conducted by Professor Redford Williams at Duke University Medical Center in the United States revealed links between high levels of hostility and the development of heart disease and other illnesses. He also found that hostile people are more likely to be smokers, to drink more alcohol, and to consume more calories—habits that are also damaging to health.

When a person becomes angry or aggressive, a series of reactions begin in the body that were once used to protect our early ancestors from the dangers of life, such as fighting a wild animal or protecting a mate. Messages are sent from the brain—specifically, the hypothalamus—to the adrenal glands, causing them to pump large amounts of adrenaline and cortisol into the bloodstream. The adrenaline makes the heart beat faster and raises blood pressure in preparation for physical activity, such as fighting or running away, while the hypothalamus stimulates a chain reaction that constricts the arteries carrying blood to the skin, kidneys, and intestines. These developments concentrate the body's reserves on immediate physical needs rather than activities like food digestion or urine processing. At the same time the hypothalamus is also instructing the arteries leading to the muscles to open wider in preparation for physical exertion.

In general, the situations that make us angry today lack the physical danger our ancestors experienced. This means that the body's reactions to anger, the increases in hormones and chemicals, are not used up in physical response.

The lack of physical action means that as blood pressure increases, the delicate lining of the arteries becomes at increased risk for being damaged by the high flow of blood passing through. Meanwhile, the adrenaline in the body stimulates fat cells to empty into the bloodstream to provide extra energy for action. The sedentary body does not burn up the fat, however, and it is sent on to the liver and converted into cholesterol. Some of the excess cholesterol in the bloodstream finds its way to the injury on the artery wall and comes to rest. Here is the beginning of a fatty buildup in the artery that may one day lead to a heart attack.

Expressing and controlling anger

It is always important to acknowledge, accept, and respect your anger, however irrational it may appear. Shaping your anger to the situation will help make it constructive and encourage the object of your anger to listen more cooperatively. The purpose of expressing anger is to relieve internal emotional pressure, as well as to convey information and effect some change.

Self-assertion is a milder and usually more effective way of conveying criticism or explaining a problem. A quiet, calm demand for recognition, a forthright statement of your position, or insistence on your rights can help you to be taken seriously without causing offense. Self-assertion classes can teach you practical skills in avoiding rage and tears, keeping a focus on the issue and creating effective communication.

If uncontrolled anger is a problem, try to identify the underlying fear that is causing your reaction and question its validity within the present context. For example, if you are frequently angry at work, you may in fact be feeling threatened by colleagues whom you see as challenging your position. Taking positive steps to improve your relationships and performance would be a more constructive response.

ANGER RELIEF

Identifying the real causes of anger is necessary to make the emotion constructive. Not only will it put the situation into context, but it will also help you come to terms with the anger and begin to resolve it. This will ensure that you do not waste your emotions on side issues that will not relieve your anger.

The way in which you express anger is important. Saying "I feel angry about. . ." or "You make me angry when. . ." can be more productive than saying "You always. . ."

If you have difficulty in expressing anger verbally, it may be helpful to find other safe outlets for relieving your feelings. For example, screaming into a pillow, writing but not sending a furious letter, or doing something physical, like going for a run, may help.

It is important to bear in mind that long-term inwardly turned or suppressed anger is self-destructive and debilitating.

Successful self-assertion involves constantly monitoring your own behavior, thoughts, and actions and taking responsibility for their initiation and consequences. It also involves being aware that you and others have the right to

- *be treated with respect.*
- *express your own feelings and opinions.*
- *set your own priorities.*
- *ask for what you want.*
- *say "no" without feeling guilty.*
- *change your mind.*
- *make mistakes.*
- *say "I don't know," "I don't understand," or "I don't care."*
- *ask for information from experts.*

Envy and jealousy

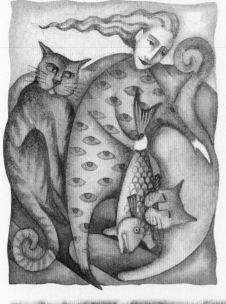

Shakespeare famously described jealousy as the "green-eyed monster," reflecting upon its destructive and threatening aspects. Understanding that fear and insecurity often lie behind jealousy and envy can help you to control such negative feelings.

The destructive path of envy and jealousy

Both envy and jealousy are forms of anxiety that usually arise from a deep-seated sense of insecurity. The main differences between the two emotions are their intensity and the target at which they are directed.

Envy is a mixture of resentment and grudging desire for the possessions, skills, or attributes of another person. It sometimes contains a highly destructive element—a wish to destroy that which is coveted but cannot be owned.

Jealousy relates solely to relationships and involves a reluctance to share someone's time and affection with others or a lack of faith in the the other person's commitment. The most common forms of jealousy involve siblings competing for parental attention, a friend refusing to accept that a companion may have other friends or interests that do not involve him or her, and partners wishing to be the sole focus of their spouse's or lover's attention. In a more general sense, a wife can be jealous of her husband's

obsession with pastimes, such as golf, fishing, or football—nonhuman but still powerful rivals for his attention, time, and energy.

Whereas envy can often be based on an objective comparison of two people's possessions or attributes, jealousy is more often a totally irrational emotion, capable of thriving even when there is no justification for it. People who feel intensely jealous in a relationship often experience feelings of obsession, over-dependency, and possessiveness. Jealousy is most often associated with loving relationships and, like possessive-ness and obsession, may be seen superficially as a romantic trait. In reality, however, all three of these emotions are destructive and preclude a genuinely healthy, loving relationship.

Jealousy not only is a highly destructive emotion, but in extreme cases can be a very dangerous one. Despite everything that a parent, friend, or partner may do to allay a jealous person's feelings,

intense emotions can build up until they turn into hostility and violence. It has been estimated that a third of domestic murders arise out of jealous feelings. In literature the best-known portrayal of this situation is in Shakespeare's play *Othello*, in which the inherent jealous traits of one person are ruthlessly exploited by another. This destructive form of morbid jealousy has come to be known as the Othello syndrome.

Allowing envy to get out of hand can also potentially cause great damage, but envy is primarily a self-destructive emotion and so usually causes more harm to the envious person than to the object of his or her resentment. Indeed, people who are the object of envy may be totally unaware that someone harbors such feelings toward them.

Both envy and jealousy can be experienced as part of a constellation of conflicting emotions. It is possible, for example, for parents to love their children, work hard to give them opportunities that they themselves never had, and be proud of their children's successes but envy them at the same time. Such ambivalence is normal and not necessarily unhealthy, but it can often be hard to admit to. Denying or repressing such feelings, however, can have destructive consequences.

"Fools may our scorn, not envy raise
For envy is a kind of praise."

JOHN GAY

The origins of envy and jealousy

Envy and jealousy often stem from a lack of parental affection in childhood. This can cause a buildup of resentment that reveals itself in an unwillingness to share a friend's time with others or envy of other people's possessions. It can also be the underlying cause of a partner's jealousy over a sexual rival.

Jealousy can also have its roots in early sibling rivalry, especially in the competition for parental love and attention. A father's irrational jealousy of his new baby, for example, may reflect a childhood experience in which he felt that the arrival of a younger sibling removed him from center stage in his parents' affections.

Envy may also arise from an inability to make inner feelings known or a lack of sufficient confidence to act on the feelings. Being envious of a friend's engagement, for example, may arise from a subconscious fear that he or she will no longer have time for you. An irrational, destructive jealousy may be fueled by low self-esteem. A person who feels physically, intellectually, and emotionally unattractive can find it difficult to accept that another's love for him or her is genuine.

A jealous person is liable to demand constant reassurance and ever more commitment and affection from the spouse, partner, or friend. Ironically, unjustified jealousy can then become self-fulfilling. The pressure of continual accusations and demands may drive a partner into a clandestine relationship, reinforcing the jealous partner's low self-esteem and increasing the desperation that he or she brings to the relationship. Indeed, jealousy can inadvertently create an atmosphere of mistrust in which individuals find it hard to develop genuine commitment.

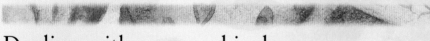

Dealing with envy and jealousy

It is perfectly normal to feel occasional pangs of jealousy or envy. We are constantly having to accept the realities of a life in which there is an unequal distribution of beauty, intelligence, wealth, health, and opportunity. Accepting these emotions is the only way to make constructive use of them.

Trying to suppress natural feelings of jealousy and envy can make these feelings harder to control. They can begin surreptitiously to influence your behavior and relationships, triggering apparently irrational actions and outbursts. If you do feel jealous or envious, try to acknowledge the feelings without being judgmental about them. By determining how appropriate your feelings are, you can begin to understand what is causing your unhappy state. Apparently irrational feelings, for example, may be the result of some unacknowledged fear or anger. A

previous failed relationship might lead to feelings of possessiveness in another relationship, or childhood deprivation might form the basis for unhealthy feelings of envy in adulthood. This form of envy needs to be confronted before it can be overcome. It is important that envious people be encouraged to start valuing themselves more highly.

Good parenting involves letting children express their jealous or envious feelings while preventing these feelings from being acted out destructively. This way, children can learn to control them.

It is important not to encourage jealous feelings in others in the mistaken belief that it is proof of their love or devotion. Neither should jealous feelings be ignored in the hope that they will subside, because too often such feelings will grow steadily more intense until they explode into uncontrolled acts of violence.

CONTROLLING ENVY AND JEALOUSY

Although jealousy and envy should not be suppressed, tight control should be kept on these feelings in order to maintain a healthy, balanced approach to relationships and keep potential emotional problems in perspective.

■ *Try to analyze why you are experiencing envy or jealousy. Are they an indication of a more deep-seated fear or insecurity, or are you simply overreacting because you have misunderstood a situation?*

■ *Avoid dwelling on the attributes, advantages, or possessions that others enjoy and that you cannot share. There are many others who are worse off than you, so be appreciative of what you have.*

■ *Make an effort to talk through the underlying cause of your jealousy with the person concerned. Explaining the reason for your fears will often help to relieve the pressure on a relationship and enable you to put it in perspective.*

■ *Remember that everybody needs to experience change and variety in order to maintain vitality in a relationship. It is important to allow a partner time to spend with friends or pursue interests and pastimes that do not involve you.*

■ *Spend time with others outside your partnership. Possessiveness leads to stagnation, whereas freedom and trust can help keep the relationship healthy, fresh, and vibrant.*

■ *Try to look at each situation from a different point of view. If you are jealous of the time that a friend or partner spends with another person, for example, think about the time that you devote to your own friends and interests.*

Fear and anxiety

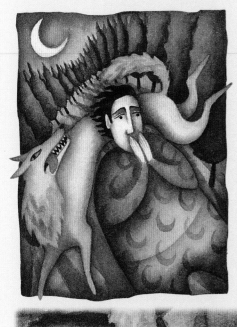

Like anger, fear and anxiety are basic emotions that are essential for our survival. We need to experience them in order to respond to a threatening situation and avoid harm. However, these emotions need to be appropriately controlled so that they don't take over your life and cause severe problems.

The difference between anxiety and fear

The words *fear* and *anxiety* are sometimes used interchangeably. More often, however, anxiety is regarded as a general feeling of apprehension and uneasiness about a situation that may have to be dealt with in the future, whereas fear usually relates to a specific and more serious threat that requires an immediate response.

Everybody experiences some degree of anxiety or fear from time to time. Anything from the threat of losing a job to moving to another town to a debilitating illness can cause feelings ranging from acute anxiety to fear.

Our bodies are programmed biologically to meet challenges with both emotional and physical responses. Anxiety or fear operates as a trigger, helping to increase alertness, clarity of thinking, and available energy so that the body can engage in self-protective action and improve its performance. The dread of an impending test or interview, a vague and unfocused concern over the thought of growing old, or anxiety about an uncertain future can all cause the familiar symptoms of a dry mouth and sweaty palms. These physical symptoms are caused by the release of the "fight or flight" hormones—adrenaline and noradrenaline—which are designed to prepare the body for a sudden burst of physical action, enabling it either to confront the threat with some action or to run away from the danger.

Although there is little point in worrying about a long-term situation that you can do nothing about, the body's responses to fear and anxiety are perfectly normal and can help you to prepare for a problem by planning practical solutions or strategies.

The uncomfortable symptoms of normal anxiety or fear disappear shortly after the task or challenge has been overcome, allowing the body to return to a calm, balanced state of equilibrium. Prolonged anxiety or fear that is not confronted and dealt with properly can cause serious problems, however. For example, free-floating anxiety that is unfocused and has little substantial cause can be self-destructive. If a person has a general sense of overwhelming anticipation but is unable to acknowledge its roots or source, the problem becomes self-perpetuating.

Another cause for concern is intense or excessive anxiety about normal activities, such as being in a crowd or using an elevator. Such trepidation can begin to inhibit a person's actions, eventually presenting social difficulties. This form of fear, usually called a phobia, often requires the professional help of a therapist or psychiatrist.

Fear and anxiety are only constructive when they are appropriate to a situation and handled in a controlled, positive manner. Both the body and mind need to recognize and respond to or dismiss the cause of anxiety in order to remain healthy and alert.

Prolonged apprehension can disrupt mental ability and alertness, inhibit concentration, and cause irritability. Unaddressed or intense anxiety can also be physically damaging. Headaches and insomnia are common physical responses that eventually accentuate the problems of poor concentration and mood swings.

"Worrying is the most natural and spontaneous of all human functions."

LEWIS THOMAS

Taking a positive approach

It is important to put fear and anxiety in perspective and understand the positive role that they play in everyday life. An appropriate concern over threatening situations ensures that we modify our behavior to avoid the consequences that may arise from unacceptable risks. For example, most people behave responsibly on the road because of a genuine fear of the consequences of driving dangerously. Those who lack this concern put themselves and other road users at risk. It is often when people are unaware of the dangers of their actions that they are most vulnerable—for example, if they fail to follow safety procedures at work because they do not understand the reasons for them.

Many people actively seek out situations that create fear in order to add excitement to their lives—the so-called adrenaline rush. The attraction of many adventure sports comes from the controlled risks that participants take. Some people also need a degree of fear and anxiety to provide a spur for accomplishing everyday tasks. Such persons are more likely to meet a work deadline or solve a difficult problem if they have a genuine concern for the possibility of failure. People who lack this concern quickly become bored, whereas those who set themselves difficult tasks and fulfill them usually gain a sense of purpose and achievement in their lives.

It is only when life's problems seem insurmountable or never ending that anxiety can lead to stress disorders, such as insomnia, headaches, stomach ulcers, tension, and depression. You should take steps to control chronic anxiety before it can affect your health. Measures include lifestyle changes to reduce stress levels, such as setting more realistic goals and managing time more efficiently to avoid unnecessary pressure.

Dealing with fear and anxiety

Anxiety or fear levels vary enormously from one individual to the next. While some people appear to sail through a crisis easily, others experience severe anxiety over the mildest of incidents. Monitoring personal fear and anxiety levels can help you assess the appropriateness of your particular response.

If fear and anxiety levels realistically reflect the level of imminent threat or challenge, it is often sensible to accept and endure the feelings. These experiences enable you to generate energy and assess what self-protective actions you can take; they also provide the basis for a suitable personal response.

If your anxiety has no positive foundation, however, or seems to be out of proportion to its cause, it may be worthwhile to consider your approach to difficult situations. Try to assess whether there is an underlying reason for such an extreme response and if there is anything you can do to help relieve it. In many cases of free-floating anxiety, it can be difficult to identify the cause. Thinking about all the different influences that currently affect your life may help you discover the underlying reasons for the anxiety. Many times it is unresolved anxieties from the past, such as being laid off from work or suffering the death of a loved one, that affect your sense of security in the present and lead to a general feeling of apprehension or despair. Even cases of mild anxiety or phobia can grow more intense and overwhelming if they are not identified and confronted at an early stage.

Everybody has worries and problems that are unique to them. Learning to identify and tackle your particular fears is a good way to feel more confident about life. Whenever you are anxious, try to assess the situation rationally and consider how appropriate your response really is.

LEARNING TO CONTROL ANXIETY

Although anxiety and fear are necessary emotions, they need to be directed into constructive responses and behavior. Out of control, they can become emotionally and physically draining, but channeled in the correct way, they can be very productive. It is always more effective to stay as calm and balanced as possible while acknowledging your inner turmoil. Directing this energy will help you put it to good use, finding solutions to the causes of your anxiety and helping you face similar situations with less fear. Below are a few tips for maintaining emotional balance and a sense of perspective.

- *The way in which you perceive a problem will be a key factor in how you react. Thinking positively always makes a situation seem less daunting.*

- *Try to reduce your anxiety by simply looking after yourself. Making a joke, telling yourself to relax, or sharing your experiences with others will help.*

- *Tell yourself that you are in control and that the situation will not get out of hand.*

- *Remember that many of the things we worry about either never happen or are not nearly as bad as they seem at first.*

- *Talk your anxieties over with other people. Independent opinions can sometimes help you to see the irrationality of a fear or provide a new perspective on coping with it.*

- *If you do feel an attack of anxiety coming on, try to calm yourself with deep breathing exercises or other relaxation techniques. (See Chapter 7 for some calming ideas.)*

Guilt

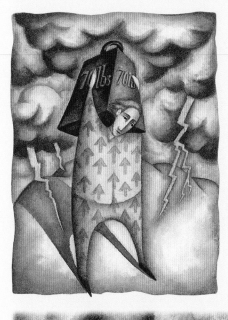

Guilt is the uncomfortable anxiety that comes from breaking established social and personal codes of moral behavior. It is an internalized experience and can often be its own form of self-criticism and punishment. Allowed to get out of control, it can become paralyzing.

What is guilt?

Guilt is a feeling connected to the concept of conscience. It relies on a coherent, personal set of moral principles that provide a reference point for distinguishing right from wrong. Historically, the ability to know right from wrong was once considered divine in origin and inherent in all human beings. A guilty conscience was actually God's voice of disapproval, and some religions still include confession and absolution as part of their practice.

Most modern thinkers, however, now generally believe that guilt develops from early childhood experiences. Parental disapproval or punishment of misbehavior sets up a system of values in which we learn right from wrong and realize the harmful effects that our actions can cause. In learning these value systems and the consequences of transgressing them, we simultaneously develop anxieties about what behaviors and attitudes are most appropriate and acceptable to society.

Although such value systems are necessary to provide social and moral codes, the discrepancy or sense of incompatibility between what we wish to do and what is conventionally "right" can be problematic. We are usually aware of what the appropriate behavior is, but we also know what we wish to do or what is of personal interest to us. In theory, of course, these concepts should never be at odds, but as everybody recognizes, in reality conflict occurs between different aspirations.

While we may always want to do what is right, numerous conflicting emotions can make right behavior difficult to identify. Guilt is the result in which we punish ourselves—an effect of the discipline and admonition we received as children or continue to receive from a religious group. Because guilt is so caught up in the conflicting emotions of love, hate, duty, and desire, we tend to turn our feelings inward, venting our frustration on ourselves.

Literature provides many examples of individuals whose guilt destroys them. One example is the Shakespearean character Lady Macbeth, who gradually disintegrates as she comes to understand the overwhelming effects of her greed and ambition. Similarly, in the novel *Thérèse Raquin* by Emile Zola, the murder of Thérèse's husband leads both the protagonist and her lover to be consumed by so much guilt that they eventually poison each other.

Few adults experience guilt in such extreme forms, and most are generally able to recognize when guilt is an appropriate form of penance. For many children, however, guilt can be an overwhelmingly powerful emotion. In very young children concepts of morality are commonly naive and only recently developed, and new concepts can often be channeled into negative self-admonition. Furthermore, the tendency to confuse fantasy with reality can sometimes lead to intense and inappropriate guilt. When a serious illness, conflict, divorce, or death occurs in a family, young children may think that their own destructive feelings or actions have caused the unhappy event. Abused children often suffer irrational guilt and feel some measure of responsibility and blame for what has been done to them.

"It is rather hard and certainly depressing to admit guilt and to repent."

HANNAH ARENDT

Aspects of guilt

Guilt can be a difficult emotion to understand and keep in perspective. Sometimes undesirable emotions, like fury, anger, or resentment, coincide with feelings of love. This can occur, for example, when caring for an elderly or ill relative. Resenting the demands placed on you by a dependent can feel very wrong, and it is often easier and more socially acceptable to endure a sense of self-admonishing guilt rather than openly expressing anger. However, in many instances honestly admitting your feelings can be helpful.

Conceding that caring for a relative at home will be difficult and discussing openly how the change in lifestyle can be best managed will be more helpful in the long term than accepting inconveniences in silent martyrdom because of feeling guilty. If self-recrimination is allowed to fester, it usually turns into further resentment and unexpressed anger.

It is always important to acknowledge your true feelings, including guilt and remorse. By ascertaining their source and assessing their appropriateness and your options, much of the self-recrimination can be relieved. If the guilt seems hugely out of scale or has no basis in reality, you may find it helpful to explore any connection between current and previous events. It may be that similar themes or circumstances are bringing up anxieties about unresolved and subconscious guilt. A naive conception of morality hanging over from childhood, for example, or discomfort about issues such as sex can cause intense feelings of guilt and further self-recrimination.

If you do feel guilty much of the time, it may be wise to seek some kind of counseling. Irrational, overwhelming, or unfocused remorse suggests that an underlying problem or cause needs to be addressed.

Is guilt a helpful emotion?

Society, for the good of the whole, sets certain standards; guilt is one tool with which it enforces them. Guilt is often an appropriate emotional response, an acknowledgment that personal behavior has harmed others. Like any tool, however, guilt can be misused to instill blind obedience and damage self-esteem and confidence. Some parents use guilt manipulatively to discipline their children, while some governments and religious groups employ a sense of inflated morality to control the populace.

Personal response to guilt determines whether it is a liberating opportunity for growth, a cunning defense, or a paralyzing trap. When guilt is appropriate to the act and results in acceptance of responsibility, atonement, and change, it is both constructive and useful. However, using guilt as a tactic—for instance, professing remorse for a destructive act but continuing to behave in the same way—is not.

This is purely a defense against facing the consequences of actions and making the effort needed to change.

Similarly, confessions of guilt can initiate insight and personal growth or simply be a way of off-loading unpleasant feelings onto someone else. While the person confessing comes out feeling emotionally clean, the recipient may be left feeling confused and mistreated. Admitting to an extramarital affair before proceeding to the next one is a particular clichéd example.

It is important to remember, though, that guilt kept in perspective is a very necessary social and personal experience. We feel guilt when we identify with the pain or injustice suffered by others or when we believe our actions to be wrong. This demonstrates that we are essentially honest and open human beings, seeing ourselves as part of a moral and considerate society.

LEARNING TO COPE WITH GUILT

While guilt may be necessary, it is important to keep it under control. To cope positively, we must learn not to accept our bad feelings at face value but examine the underlying causes. To do this, it is necessary to confront particular issues rather than abstract notions and think about how appropriate and rational your feelings and behavior really are.

- *If you feel guilty and worthless, try to evaluate what these feelings represent. What characteristics make another person worthless, and do you really meet these criteria?*

- *Consider whether you are applying the same standards to yourself as to other people. Are you being too self-critical?*

- *Maintain perspective. If you do something wrong, acknowledge it but do not consider yourself to be inherently bad.*

- *Try to understand the reason behind your actions. It may be that your initial behavior felt appropriate at the time and that the intent was good, even if the outcome was not.*

- *If you do suffer from excessive guilt, think about what might be causing your behavior and feelings. Could an unresolved problem from the past be affecting your judgment?*

- *Talk to other people about your feelings. As a common side effect of bereavement, anger, or love, guilt needs to be expressed in the open rather than internalized into self-recrimination.*

- *Accept that you can't be perfect. While we should all try to make life as pleasurable as possible for ourselves and others, remember that you are human and things are never really black or white.*

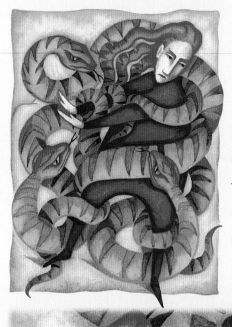

Hatred and disgust

Despite the negative aspects of hatred and disgust, everybody suffers from these feelings from time to time. While it may be difficult to see the positive elements of these emotions, their presence should be acknowledged in order to deal with them constructively.

The politics of hatred and disgust

The terms *hate* and *disgust* are sometimes used interchangeably, but they actually describe two different things. Hatred is usually directed toward a person or group of people, whereas disgust tends to describe feelings about a characteristic or event. We may feel an intense sense of dislike, or hatred, for a person who has treated us badly in the past, and that feeling may have festered through unresolved anger and frustration. On the other hand, we might feel disgust at the behavior of someone we don't even know personally. In fact, disgust often contains an element of moral judgment and physical aversion. We tend to be disgusted by those things that we find personally offensive or that we have learned to regard as morally or socially reprehensible. Cases of social injustice, such as racism or the exclusion of certain people from the benefits and rights granted to the broader society,

may engender deep feelings of loathing. Indeed, actions that affect or harm innocent or vulnerable persons, such as pedophilia or the abuse of old people, can cause very strong sensations of revulsion and disgust. Our objections and aversion to such behaviors derive from the values and morals that we acquire as children. As our parents express their disapproval of certain conduct, we learn a set of values that we keep and develop throughout life.

Social evolution also helps us to revise these principles. As society changes its concept of right and wrong, individuals learn to regard some behaviors with a new sense of disgust or acceptance. Opinions on the acceptability of imperialism, for example, changed quite dramatically during the 20th century, while race discrimination—once tolerated in many societies—was gradually rejected, in theory if not

entirely in practice, by many governments and communities in the Western world. Moral judgments can become more or less liberal. Open discussion of sex and sexuality, for instance, was once viewed with disapproval but is now more accepted.

Hatred is usually more personal in nature and is often a natural defense against other painful emotions. When we feel powerless, angry, or rejected, we tend to channel these feelings into a form of hatred. We may claim to hate the person who has rejected us or express hatred of a certain situation in which we find ourselves. For this reason hatred is often associated with the apparently opposing emotion of love. When we are emotionally vulnerable, we often suffer from a low sense of self-esteem and channel these negative feelings into more intense responses.

Rejection in love can overwhelm a person to the point where rational objectivity seems impossible and hatred becomes the main means of release. However, the opposite of love is not really hatred but indifference. A lack of emotional energy is far more destructive to both the individual and the recipient than controlled acknowledgment of emotion. Both hatred and disgust at least indicate passionate interest.

"If you hate a person, you hate something in him that is part of yourself. What isn't part of ourselves doesn't disturb us."

HERMANN HESSE

Hatred and anger

Although it is possible to identify the different circumstances in which hatred and disgust often arise, the causes of such profound emotions can often be more complex. The notion of hatred, for example, is a mixed one for many people. We tend to use the term quite loosely, describing something or somebody that we dislike or are unhappy with as an object of hate. In fact, hate is actually a very intense sensation and less common than you might think. Claiming to hate somebody at work, for example, normally describes a dislike of his or her behavior and attitude, rather than an intense abhorrence of that person. Genuine hatred is normally the product of prolonged and unexpressed anger that festers inside, becoming increasingly poisonous and destructive. It assumes a certain amount of premeditation, not the immediate, disgruntled response to a situation but accumulative anger and displeasure that stays with you. For this reason, it is important to address your anger correctly (see page 81) in order to prevent it from becoming negatively and dangerously unfocused.

Interestingly, such distinction is reflected in the approach of the law to violent crime. Those offenses committed in a moment of passionate anger are often looked upon more sympathetically than those committed after cool, rational premeditation. It seems that while society considers anger to be a dangerous state, hatred is looked on as the more socially reprehensible expression.

The inner self

The most damaging aspects of both disgust and hatred occur when they are turned inward on the self. They can affect confidence and self-esteem, undermining how you feel about yourself and about the world around you. Self-hatred is often linked with depression. It can be common to feel unhappy with aspects of your life while believing that things are beyond your control; this in turn leads to a sense of self-loathing.

Questioning your own behavior while refusing to address the cause of the problem can lead to a profound sense of self-disappointment and frustration. You may feel angry, for example, at not enjoying rapid progress in your career but choose to reprimand yourself for failure rather than discuss your problems at work or do something about them. Or you may hate the way you talk and behave with others and yet feel unable to break the chain of conduct. Such self-hatred merely increases low self-esteem and lack of confidence.

Similarly, inappropriate disgust tends to reflect an unresolved problem with the self rather than a valued moral judgment. Many of these cases reflect a difficulty in coming to terms with one's individuality. Subconscious fears, for which a person actually identifies some similarity between himself and the object of disgust, can often cause intense feelings. A woman repulsed by any reference to sex, for example, may well have unresolved feelings about her own sexuality.

In the case of both hatred and disgust, therefore, it is important to maintain a sense of self-esteem. Try to isolate dissatisfaction with any aspects of your behavior or attitudes from your basic faith in yourself as a person. We can all make changes in our beliefs or behavior; in fact, this effort shows that we have the capacity to grow and evolve. Unhappiness with an aspect of yourself can be a catalyst for positive change; it need never turn into self-hatred.

STEPS TO OVERCOME SELF-HATRED

Imperfection is an inherent part of being human, and we can all identify aspects of ourselves with which we are not entirely happy. Such minor displeasure should never be allowed to evolve into full self-hatred, however. There are a number of steps you can take to help yourself channel self-criticism into a more constructive perspective. Assessing how you really feel about yourself can provide the necessary insight to spur emotional growth.

- *Accept the impossibility of perfection. Carefully distinguishing between characteristics of yourself that potentially can be improved and those that cannot will enable you to react to events in a more rational way.*

- *Try to work on areas that can be improved. Some of the visualization exercises featured in this book can help to raise self-esteem, as well as promote relaxation.*

- *Explore the internalized standards against which you measure yourself. Some may be personally relevant, but others may be unrealistic and not constructive.*

- *Treat yourself to something special occasionally and learn to focus on your personal worth. Buying yourself some new clothes or spending some time pursuing a favorite activity will help you reinforce your self-perception and come to terms with who you really are. Although everyone can improve in some areas, constant self-castigation will only demoralize your spirits.*

- *Remember that everybody has something good to offer, and hating yourself will only undermine your positive qualities.*

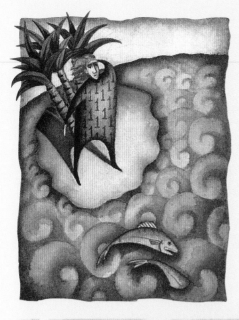

Loneliness

Unlike the feelings of guilt, envy, and jealousy, loneliness is not the subject of finely tuned definitions or complex theories of origin. Yet feeling lonely—isolated, estranged from others, or companionless—is a universal experience and an inherent part of human life.

Loneliness and being alone

Everybody experiences loneliness sometimes. Occasional bouts can actually be quite healthy, encouraging us to identify those parts of our lives that we really enjoy or yearn for. Without experiencing solitude, we would be unable to appreciate the comfort and support of a loving social network. In fact, emotional maturity largely involves the capacity to be alone. As young children we learn to go off and explore, develop our skills, and investigate new experiences, all the time knowing that our parents or caregivers are still there, offering support, comfort, and love. This is perhaps one of the fundamental differences between feeling lonely and being alone.

While many people enjoy moments of solitude, conscious of the available support network provided by friends and family, others find being alone a rather intense and saddening experience. It is possible to experience acute loneliness while surrounded by close friends or family members. There are many people who have very active work and social lives and still feel that something fundamental is missing, that deep down they are both lonely and insecure. One common cause of such angst is the absence of a partner. It is not unusual for unmarried people to feel that they should or would like to share their lives with a single key person and that no amount of daily socializing will ever fill this apparent gap.

A bereavement, separation, or sense of disorder can also cause painful self-questioning and solitude. For this reason loneliness is often a derivative of other profound emotions and experiences. Social protocol, together with anger, jealousy, or unrequited love, can help contribute to an individual's experiences of isolation and loneliness.

Most discomfort with solitude is brought on by a combination of circumstances. Feeling ostracized or like an outsider—for example, being gay in a predominantly heterosexual environment or being in a strange city alone—can lead to feelings of loneliness and despair. Hierarchies at work can be particularly isolating when managers and their subordinates allow class and financial circumstances to define further boundaries. Unemployment, single parenthood, or rural surroundings can also foster feelings of unwanted solitude. Essentially, loneliness is brought on by an inability to establish contacts and relationships, perhaps as a result of constant changing of jobs or the inability to relate to people around us.

Personality traits, in addition to circumstances, can also contribute to loneliness. While one widow may find the strength to rebuild a social network, for example, another may remain forever lonely and isolated. Every individual's tendency toward emotional isolation varies, and there is always a set of circumstances—ranging from geography to personal disposition—that helps to determine how well a person copes with being alone. Childhood experiences, as well as those of adult life, affect how often a person is and feels alone. Even denying yourself open expression of emotion can lead to feelings of isolation in which it seems that nobody can identify with your hurt.

"I love tranquil solitude,
And such society, as is quiet, wise, and good."

PERCY BYSSHE SHELLEY

Being alone and happy

The capacity to be alone and contented develops from early childhood experiences. Repeated separations from our mothers usually help us to build up a sense of security in which we can feel comfortable with the idea of being alone. As we learn to tolerate separation and solitude, we become more resourceful and independent, confident in our own abilities, and better prepared for the realities of later life.

In adulthood, being alone can be a welcome, refreshing relief from the stresses and demands of interacting constantly with others. Solitude provides the opportunity to rest and replenish emotional resources before returning to the world of professional, social, or family relationships. It can also be a time of immense creativity. Many of the great works of literature, art, and music have been produced within the peaceful parameters of solitude, and some of today's artists still retire from busy social interaction when they wish to focus on their work. The American author Henry David Thoreau (1817–1862) famously wrote about the virtues of his solitary existence in *Walden, or Life in the Woods.* Pursuing a hermitlike lifestyle for several months, Thoreau lived in a cabin near Walden Pond, in Massachusetts, and wrote several books, including an account of his own experiences there.

The difference between being solitary and lonely and being solitary and content depends on several factors. These include whether solitude is voluntary or imposed and whether it is within personal control. If you are able to determine just how and when you are alone, it is possible to cherish these moments. Indeed, solitude offers the perfect opportunity to get to know your true self better and can be a path to greater happiness.

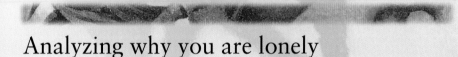

Analyzing why you are lonely

If you are feeling lonely, think about what could be causing this despondency. Consider whether you feel lonely when you are keeping your own company only or whether you have a general sense of isolation, even when you are surrounded by people. Thinking about when and where you get these feelings can help you to identify the situations that are influencing you.

If your feelings of loneliness seem to be out of proportion to your social life, it is worth considering how healthy your self-esteem is. Many people become depressed and lonely because they no longer feel capable of coping on their own, losing confidence in their abilities and thus yearning for the distraction of company and support of others. Such low self-esteem can then become cyclical because sufferers increasingly see occasional moments of solitude as accentuated periods of isolation. Instead of craving some solitude, they focus on the negative elements, often feeling outcast, lonely, and rejected.

If you do feel lonely much of the time, it may be worth trying to increase your interaction with others. This does not mean abandoning important moments of solitude but simply using the time when you are in company to build your self-esteem and perception. By paying special attention to listening, interacting, and empathizing with others, you can actually help raise your own sense of self-worth, which will provide you with the confidence to believe in your value as both an interactive member of society and as a single person. By feeling self-assured, adequate, and fulfilled, you set up a good basis for establishing relationships with others who will value you. It is worth remembering that those people who have trouble accepting themselves are often the loneliest.

LEARNING TO COPE WITH LONELINESS

Although solitude can be a rewarding and revitalizing time, it is important not to let such periods develop into sensations of acute loneliness. If you do find that loneliness starts to take over your life, think about some positive ways in which you can improve your self-esteem. (Chapter 3 includes some ideas.) Being open to change is necessary in order to assess and then address those areas of your life that cause you to feel lonely or miserable. Loneliness is part of the condition of being human, but it needn't be self-destructive.

■ *Readjust your expectations of yourself and others. Remember that everybody experiences the same feelings as you do sometimes, and offering sympathy and company is a good way to set up a support structure for yourself.*

■ *Take advantage of but do not abuse the comfort and help offered by your friends and family.*

■ *Learn to focus on, listen to, and respond to others. Deliberately increasing social contact is another strategy for combating loneliness, but this will be beneficial only when any issues of self-worth have been resolved.*

■ *Consider taking up a new hobby or activity that will broaden your range of experiences, interaction, and expectations.*

■ *Remember the value of occasional peaceful solitude. It not only offers an opportunity to recharge your batteries but can also be a period of creativity.*

■ *When you do feel lonely, channel the energy into positive actions that reinforce self-esteem and help you to believe in your self-worth and your ability to cope.*

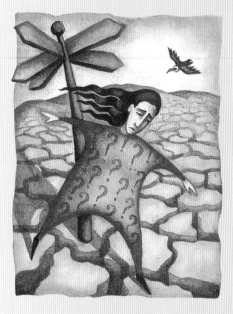

Emotional insecurity

The occasional feeling of insecurity is a perfectly normal condition, but when it is constant and has no obvious cause, it can be a highly destructive emotion. Insecurity can interfere with normal social interaction and make it very difficult to form lasting, meaningful relationships.

Insecurity as a barrier to relationships

Emotional insecurity is a general term for a low sense of self-esteem and of emotional self-assurance. Individuals who constantly experience it feel anxious and vulnerable, and they lack confidence, particularly in their social skills and ability to interact with others.

A degree of emotional insecurity is a normal part of life and is the typical reaction to sudden, destabilizing life events, such as the loss of a job or the breakdown of a relationship. Intense, pervasive, and long-lasting emotional insecurity, however, with no obvious external cause, is a much more serious problem and in many cases may have a deep-rooted psychological cause, perhaps stemming from childhood experiences. Whether emotional insecurity represents a serious problem depends on its intensity, or degree.

Deep-seated emotional insecurity is often linked to innate feelings of guilt, inadequacy, or inferiority. It can distort an individual's perceptions of reality and adversely affect the way he or she is able to relate to others on a daily basis. In turn, this will create a barrier to the development of committed long-term relationships.

Emotional insecurity can manifest itself in many different ways. Forming a series of premature, indiscriminate, idealized attachments is often a sign of both emotional insecurity and immaturity. An insecure person's desperate need for constant reassurance can cause the object of his or her affection to feel suffocated and overburdened and to begin withdrawing from the relationship. This behavior, in turn, intensifies the insecure person's emotional state.

Many insecure people try to hide their vulnerability by being excessively self-reliant and independent, thus sabotaging any potential attachment before it has a chance to develop. Other people may resort to destructive social behavior, such as bullying or acting in a brash, loud-mouthed, or overbearing manner.

Compulsive caregiving is another subconscious self-defense strategy employed by insecure people, especially women. By choosing an even less emotionally secure person to love and care for, the caregiver's own fragile position is bolstered in comparison.

In some cases an individual's emotional insecurity reveals itself in an obsessive dedication to a career or a vocation such as charitable work. These individuals, often known as workaholics, are attempting to prove to themselves that they are both worthy and valued by others. The amount of time and effort that the workaholic spends on his or her job or vocation also provides a subconscious excuse for failing to devote a similar amount of time and energy to maintaining a relationship. While it is true that some people lead full, productive lives without experiencing close emotional attachments, their contentedness still depends on feeling secure. For others, having a reliable, sympathetic witness to their thoughts and feelings and an emotional reference point during times of crisis or self-doubt is a prerequisite to feeling emotionally complete. Regardless of your marital status, having long-established platonic friendships or strong family ties can contribute to such security.

"It is a miserable state of mind to have few things to desire and many things to fear."

FRANCIS BACON

The roots of emotional insecurity

Extreme emotional insecurity is thought to have its roots in the mother-infant relationship. A lack of maternal affection or being subjected to constant criticism can instill in a child the innate feeling that he or she is not worthy of love and attention and not important enough to be able to guarantee the mother's continued presence.

As the child grows up, this insecurity and lack of self-worth continually blocks his or her ability to interact with others. The individual lacks the confidence to form a relationship or is unable to accept that any relationship is dependable.

In a successful mother-infant relationship, the mother helps her child to know that he or she is loved and valued, regardless of faults, mistakes, and imperfections. This helps to establish an emotional environment in which the youngster feels increasingly secure and certain that the mother's absences are only temporary. Eventually, this sense of self-worth becomes internalized and establishes in the child the confidence that the mother will always return. The growing infant can use this secure emotional base as the springboard from which to explore various forms of social interaction. During adolescence and adulthood, the individual's sense of worth provides both the confidence to seek out close emotional ties and the security to believe that they will last.

Dramatic changes in life can also undermine emotional security. For example, it is natural to derive your identity, at least in part, from the roles of others, such as a spouse, partner, parent, or professional mentor. If a "role player" goes away, especially if unexpectedly or unjustly, a cocktail of powerful emotions may be released, including hurt, anger, and depression, and lead to an identity crisis with an acute loss of the sense of self.

Building emotional security

The crises that occur in everyone's life from time to time can also provide opportunities for change and advancement, although that may be difficult to accept at the time, The ending of a disastrous relationship may be an opportunity for reflection, emotional growth, and insight, and perhaps help you to make a more suitable choice of partner next time. Similarly, the unexpected loss of your job may pave the way for a rejuvenating career change. Experiencing emotional insecurity can also help you to develop compassion and understanding for the problems and emotional crises of others.

It is important to feel confident in your own emotional resources and your ability to cope with whatever challenges life may present. Working through and coming to terms with your unfulfilled emotional potential is an important part of becoming a more mature individual.

Take an objective look at your emotional background, particularly your childhood, because it can help you to understand and deal with the origins of any current emotional insecurity. Explore any feelings that seem inappropriate or exaggerated, such as extreme reactions to petty mistakes made by a friend or partner. They may relate to an unresolved problem in your past or in the relationship itself that needs to be addressed. Try not to have unrealistic expectations of yourself, others, or a relationship. Rather than striving for perfection, accept the concept of something being good enough.

If emotional insecurity is seriously affecting your life and relationships, consider getting counseling or psychotherapy. Both can help you build emotional self-confidence and thus offer a sensible investment in your future well-being, as well as that of the present.

WAYS TO RESTORE YOUR SENSE OF SELF-WORTH

It is easier to restore a healthy sense of self-worth that has suffered a temporary blow than to try to establish it where little or none existed before. While the following suggestions can help in many cases, for some people it may be worth considering professional help.

- *Accept that some emotional insecurity is the appropriate response to a crisis and not a sign of weakness.*

- *Give yourself credit for having coped with a crisis and remind yourself, repeatedly if necessary, of your good points.*

- *Try not to overidentify with one aspect of your life; remember that you are multifaceted.*

- *If you experience rejection by a partner or employer, try to remember that nothing has changed about you and that you are still the same person.*

- *Give yourself time; don't feel guilty for not having restored your self-confidence according to an unrealistic self-imposed schedule.*

- *Accept that having ambivalent or contradictory feelings about another person is a normal and healthy part of a relationship.*

- *Try to make an objective assessment of the scale, timing, and intensity of your emotional insecurity in relation to present events. If they are exaggerated, consider seeking professional help.*

- *Look after yourself; eat well, get adequate sleep, and exercise regularly.*

- *Learn new skills or take up new interests or pastimes.*

- *Admit your suffering to others whom you trust, and accept their compassion and support.*

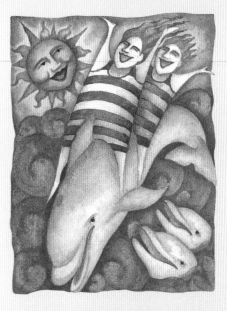

Happiness

Love, success, and a general sense of well-being contribute to an individual's contentment, but it is not necessary to enjoy all of these to feel generally happy. Happiness can range from passive serenity to wild excitement, from overwhelming passion to quiet, internal peace.

The quest for happiness

Ask people about their main ambition in life, and most will claim that they simply want to be happy. Happiness is seen by many as the purpose of existence, the reason for enduring the tribulations of daily life. Feeling content with ourselves and our lives provides the inspiration to go on and meet new challenges, face the trivialities of routine, and pursue different experiences.

The majority of people would agree that happiness is part of the essence of being. Success in love, work, and relationships depends on feeling content with both yourself and those around you, and you can begin to understand and relate to others only when you are truly content within yourself.

Despite this assessment, everybody has moments in which they believe that they could be happier or more fulfilled. We spend our lives seeking further contentment, believing that the next promotion, material acquisition, or relationship will help us feel more complete, and sometimes these very desires are a source of discontent.

Many religions are founded on the idea that essential happiness and reward come through continually striving to be better. Christian doctrine, for example, asserts the role of virtue and social morality, suggesting that internal contentment comes through communal responsibility and focusing on the spiritual aspects of life. Many Eastern philosophies, on the other hand, teach the importance of self-contemplation and individuality. While still asserting the importance of society, Buddhism and Taoism suggest that individuals have the ability to control their own sense of happiness. They posit that it is through striving for self-fulfillment that we become valuable, sharing, and essentially happy human beings.

The problem is, of course, that happiness is essentially a subjective experience. We each have our own expectations of life, our aspirations for the future, and our own natural dispositions. While some people are content with maintaining a simple and secure lifestyle, others require more,

believing that a change in routine or the acquisition of prestigious material objects will enhance their contentment.

Many individuals equate personal happiness with wealth, power, or fame, while others view wealth as an encumbrance and base happiness on inner, spiritual peace. Even sexual fulfillment can be seen as a major criterion of contentment or as a symbol of sensual needs that should be minimized for greater spiritual happiness.

As we gain maturity, we tend to change our expectations and requirements. Infants are generally content with warmth, food, love, and comfort. A young adult's sense of happiness, however, may come from the sudden freedom and opportunities offered by adulthood. A middle-aged person's happiness may come from a growing family, while for many older people, happiness comes from maintaining independence and enjoying the fruits of an active younger life. Similarly, those things that diminish our sense of happiness can be just as varied. Lack of support, independence, company, or wealth can inhibit contentment, and so it is important to set realistic expectations. Most people find that simply enjoying a sense of control is one of the best routes to self-esteem and self-fulfillment.

"The days that make us happy make us wise."

JOHN MASEFIELD

94

The natural high

Although external events, such as falling in love or suffering a serious injury or loss, can affect your level of happiness temporarily, there is evidence to suggest that most people eventually return to their own basic level of contentment. We all have our own individual threshold, a natural set of expectations and emotional desires that remains fairly consistent throughout life.

When we feel moments of occasional elation, however, it is because external events can temporarily disrupt this equilibrium, bringing intense sensations of joy and happiness. As human beings we naturally seek out the factors that can contribute to such feelings. Sharing a joke, for example, pursuing a favorite activity, or enjoying the company of others all provide moments of additional happiness—periods in which we are even more content than usual and during which we feel complete.

Scientists now believe that there is actually a physiological basis for the sensations experienced in such moments. Natural chemicals called endorphins, which are produced by the pituitary gland in the brain, help both to minimize pain and to improve feelings of well-being. These chemicals help to control the body's responses to stress and to intensify positive feelings. Exercise is particularly associated with increasing the number of endorphins produced, which explains why many athletes feel what they describe as a natural high after a long workout. Endorphins are released even after moderate exercise, which is a good argument for the benefits of getting fit. Even laughter can be responsible for producing these chemicals, which probably explains why we often feel so much better after sharing a good laugh with friends.

The middle way

Although most people have their own basic level of happiness, it is possible to improve and develop this threshold. By avoiding violent swings between depression and elation, for example, you can find the middle path—a sensible balance between the need for instant gratification and selfless postponement of pleasure. Most of us feel that we could be happier at least some of the time, and setting up the right circumstances and frame of mind can help to make periods of contentment more prolonged and fulfilling.

One psychologist, Michael Fordyce, believes that you can improve your sense of happiness simply by increasing the frequency of positive emotions rather than by aiming for major changes in your life. This can be achieved by following a number of different steps that provide the right support network and basis. Strengthening your personal

relationships, for example, will help to make daily life easier and encourage you to value and accept other people's ideas and attitudes. Similarly, setting up a series of personal aims that keep you busy and help you avoid boredom can provide a sense of achievement. Opting for meaningful activities or work can be particularly rewarding, but if this is difficult to achieve, finding hobbies that are stimulating can be fulfilling too.

It is interesting to note that many people who report high levels of happiness tend to lead sociable, outgoing lives. Encouraging yourself to make new contacts and friends can be beneficial for both work and social opportunities.

Although no miracle change will occur overnight, it is possible to provide yourself a better grounding so that you enjoy moments of happiness to their fullest. You may even find that your basic level of happiness improves.

ENHANCING YOUR LEVEL OF HAPPINESS

It is important to remember that like all emotions, happiness is a question of balance. Nobody can remain in an intense state of elation all the time—just as nobody should feel miserable for too long. If you do feel that your personal level of happiness needs improving, take a look at your current situation and try to assess what is missing. Rather than looking at extremes, try to find the small imbalances and address them gradually. In addition to the suggestions offered by Michael Fordyce (see below, left) there are simple, practical things you can do to improve your general outlook.

■ *Consider the benefits of your personal pleasures. While some activities, such as listening to or performing music, are harmless, others, like chocolate and alcohol, need to be enjoyed in moderation, or they may damage your health and your self-esteem.*

■ *Do moderate exercise on a regular basis; it will not only improve your well-being but also provide the natural benefits of endorphins. Taking up a physical activity can also help you to meet new friends and relieve much of the stress that inhibits happiness.*

■ *Try to live in the present rather than worrying about either the past or future. Face reality with an open mind, and if you must anticipate problematic events, use this concern to channel your energies into constructive preparation.*

■ *Cultivate a sense of humor; it will help you to remain positive and make others more sympathetic to your situation. Trying to see the funny side of a situation will also help you to take yourself a little less seriously.*

ACHIEVING BALANCE

Coming to terms with all your emotions is by far the best way to achieve a sense of balance, although keeping conflicting feelings under control can be difficult.

Everybody differs in temperament, but there are a few things we can all do to make coming to terms with the self easier. By achieving personal insight, you can open yourself more to other people and make relationships and daily interactions flow more smoothly. As an individual you will always be slightly different from everybody else. This knowledge should be used to work in your favor, making you feel unique and special rather than self-conscious and uncomfortable.

We all have our faults as well as good qualities, and learning to identify and acknowledge them can help us to attain a greater sense of self-esteem. For this reason it is important to accept and respect all of your feelings, even the ones that you consider to be negative, such as anger, guilt, or depression. These emotions are an inherent part of you and need to be acknowledged rather than denied. Try to see them as a first step toward self-enlightenment, a realization of who you really are and the value of your true worth.

There will always be times when you react inappropriately to a situation or feel your emotions getting out of control. In certain situations—falling in love, for instance—excessive sensations can be pleasurable, but the letdown if the relationship fails can be even more intense. In the same vein, confronting yourself with unnecessary guilt or hatred can lead to self-recrimination and pain. It is important to try to keep a balanced perspective. Enjoy moments of elation or passion but remember that excessive sadness or anger is of little use to anybody. When you do feel a rush of emotion, try to channel the energy constructively, and keep in mind that no one feeling, whether it's joy or profound sadness, lasts forever.

It is best to seek the middle path between personal abilities and ambition. We all need aspirations, yet we must still exist within our own limitations. These boundaries, just like our successes, are a part of us and they reinforce the concept that we must accept and like every part of ourselves in order to be emotionally healthy.

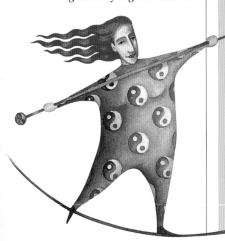

WALKING THE TIGHT ROPE
When you feel yourself becoming emotionally overwrought, try to sit back calmly, relax, and reestablish emotional balance. Be as objective as possible and take deep breaths to help yourself gradually regain control.

ACHIEVING BALANCE IN YOUR RELATIONSHIPS

Achieving balance often involves walking a fine line between powerful emotions. This is easier said than done, however, especially if you often feel insecure. Taking the time to relate to other people will help you to think about how you communicate your own emotions and to feel better understood. Think about how you see yourself, as well as how you view others.

▶ *Consider how receptive you are to other people's emotions. You deserve the same level of patience, understanding, and support that you offer your friends.*

▶ *Actively seek out companionship and support networks. This does not mean you believe that you are emotionally complete only in the presence of others, but that you value the fresh perspectives and intimacy of a range of different types of relationships.*

▶ *If you would like to share your life with someone but are currently single, don't allow yourself to become depressed. Focus instead on other areas of your life, encouraging the development of other fulfilling relationships.*

▶ *All of us need to feel that we can be emotionally open and honest. Providing emotional support to other people will help you feel more complete within yourself.*

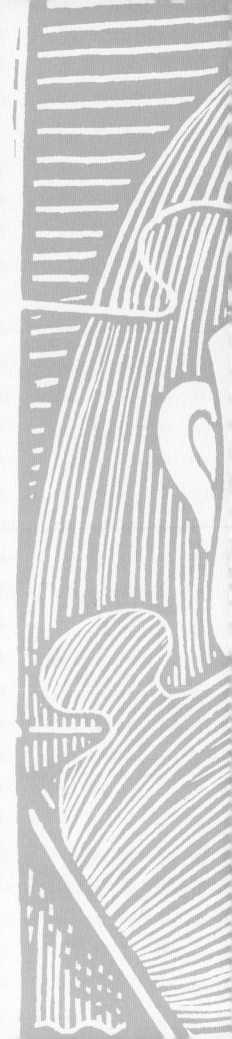

CHAPTER 5

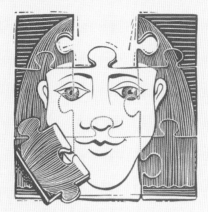

SERIOUS EMOTIONAL PROBLEMS

*We can do much to maintain and improve
our own emotional health and to support the
mental health of our loved ones, but things may go
wrong occasionally. There are a number of disorders
that can upset emotional balance. Understanding
the symptoms and causes of such conditions
can aid in dealing with their effects.*

DEPRESSION

Everybody has transient periods of feeling sad or not quite right. Depression, however, is a condition in which people feel profound unhappiness for much of the time.

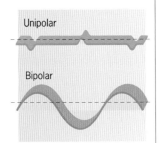

MOOD SWINGS
A sufferer of unipolar depression experiences a fairly stable pattern of depressed mood. In contrast, a sufferer of bipolar depression has extreme mood swings.

Depression—feeling down or sad—is experienced by everyone from time to time. This state of mind is called reactive depression, and it is usually a response to an event, such as the death of a loved one or the loss of a job. But when periods of unhappiness are intense and enduring, depression is considered a serious mood disorder. It has two major forms: unipolar and bipolar.

Unipolar depression, also called clinical depression or major depression, is the most common type; it can range from mild (called dysthemia) to severe and has a number of symptoms (see right), but the sufferer's mood remains relatively stable, perhaps punctuated only occasionally by periods of more benign moods.

Bipolar depression, or manic depression as it is more commonly known, involves extreme alternations in mood. Periods of depression are interspersed with episodes of mania in which the individual is extremely energetic, elated, and hyperactive. Each mood can last for days or even weeks and is exhausting because the person must adjust physically and mentally to its demands. Most sufferers don't realize what is actually happening to them, and they find both states equally taxing and bewildering.

UNIPOLAR DEPRESSION

Unipolar depression is the most common of all psychological problems, with an estimated 10 percent of the developed world's population suffering from it at any given time. It has a number of symptoms, including overall depressed mood, poor self-image, inappropriate feelings of guilt, pessimism, sleep disorders (insomnia or an excessive sleep habit), poor ability to concentrate, loss of interest in favorite activities, lethargy or hyperactivity, major weight loss or gain, and, in severe cases, persistent thoughts of suicide. A patient is considered clinically depressed when at least five of the above symptoms have been present for a month.

Large-scale events that have no direct relevance to the individual can accentuate a depressed person's sadness. Famine or war in another country, for example, can feel like a personal problem and intensify the worrying and sense of despair. Many effects of depression are interconnected. While a sufferer may experience a lack of interest in sex, for example, this disinterest may be caused either by the depression itself or by the low self-esteem that depression incurs. Poor memory, which is experienced by some depressed people, is frequently caused by fatigue and a lack of motivation to remember significant moments or events.

Anxiety is often a common symptom of depression because an event that can trigger it, such as losing a job or loved one or important relationship, can then set up a

MOOD DISORDERS AND ARTISTIC GENIUS

Mood disorders tend to be especially common in people who are creative, and many researchers believe there is some kind of biochemical link with the artistic temperament. Many famous writers, painters, and musicians have suffered from depression; the writers Virginia Woolf, Sylvia Plath, and Ernest Hemingway all had severe spells. While depression is not a necessary criterion for creativity, it does seem that many sufferers are able to channel their negative energies into positive achievements.

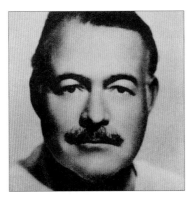

ERNEST HEMINGWAY
The Hemingway family has a history of depression, which has led to five suicides, including that of the famous novelist himself.

fear of similar incidences. As anxiety becomes constant, insomnia or poor ability to concentrate may occur, thus leading to further depression and self-recrimination. The perpetual cycle of these emotions is the reason so many people find it difficult to lift their own mood and escape from depression. A depressed mood can affect behavior as well, often manifesting itself in persistent irritability, impatience, and unreasonable outbursts of anger.

How depression occurs

There are many causes of depression, and there is considerable debate over which aspects are the most significant. Some clinicians argue that depression is largely genetic and is precipitated by factors already present at birth. Others believe that childhood experiences or recent disturbing life events in adulthood are the main causes.

The traditional psychoanalytic view of depression, first proposed by psychiatrist Sigmund Freud, suggests that depression results from the way people react to a real or imagined loss. Freud argued that some individuals respond to loss by regressing to an earlier emotional period. Losing a loved one, for instance, might cause a person to turn earlier feelings of unexpressed anger against the self in a process called introjection. Freud believed that all forms of depression were a variation on this single theme, and though his theories have generated controversy, they are still influential in modern psychotherapy.

DID YOU KNOW?
People who lose their spouses through divorce are more likely to suffer depression than those who lose them through death. There are many reasons for this, but one key factor may be that social networks are often at their strongest during bereavement. After a divorce, however, people may find themselves drifting away from or even in conflict with the friends and family members who would ordinarily be there for them.

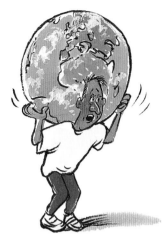

BEARING THE WEIGHT OF THE WORLD
Although it can be common to feel the world's problems intensely when you're depressed, it is necessary to keep a sense of proportion about external events.

BE KIND TO YOURSELF

Many people with depression experience such low self-esteem that they punish themselves for their lethargy and general unhappiness. In fact, the best thing people can do if they are feeling low is to start being a little kinder to themselves. Just as you look after yourself during physical illness, you should try to accept that you need extra attention and self-care if you are having emotional problems.

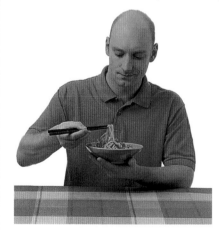

MAKE SURE YOU EAT WELL
Many depressed people starve or gorge themselves, hating their lack of self-control and punishing themselves. It's a good idea to prepare yourself small portions of nourishing and attractive food at certain times of the day—no matter what your appetite dictates.

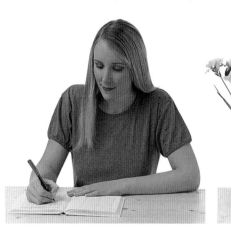

KEEP A DIARY
Taking note of daily achievements and positive experiences, however modest, is a constructive way of learning to feel good about yourself. Making daily affirmations (see page 149) may help you to focus your attention on the positive side of life.

INVOLVE YOURSELF
Concentrate on the present rather than being obsessed with the past or future. Taking the time to develop a hobby or direct your attention to something productive will help you to reconnect the self with a sense of worth and purpose.

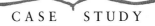
A Depressed Husband

Depression can be caused by a whole range of factors, but whatever the trigger, its effects can be severe. Learning to cope with a new set of restrictions on your life, such as those imposed by disability, can be particularly trying. Individuals with such problems often become so consumed with guilt and low self-esteem that they lose all of their vital energy and enthusiasm.

Steve is 35 and married to Jen. Two years ago he was involved in an automobile accident that left him with back pain that is serious enough to be disabling at times. Although he did receive compensation, he had to give up working as a fireman. The wrench of losing a career he loved has been made worse by the fact that Steve hasn't been able to find any other work.

Everyone has been sympathetic to Steve, but he hates feeling so dependent and having to rely on his wife's income. His inability to work and the guilt he feels from it are now feeding his lethargy, and he has lost interest in going out or socializing. Steve thinks that he is a burden on everybody, and he has become seriously depressed.

WHAT SHOULD STEVE DO?

Although Steve received counseling immediately after the accident, he now needs further therapy to help him deal with the problems that have subsequently arisen. Speaking to a therapist about how he feels could enable him to see that his low self-esteem is causing him to feel guilty and depressed. Steve knows that people wish to help him, and he has to overcome his pride and sense of self-recrimination.

Steve should think about contacting an agency that finds work specifically for people with some kind of disability. Contributing to the family income again would help to improve his self-esteem and mood and mitigate some of the boredom and lethargy he feels.

Action Plan

FAMILY
Take time to talk to Jen and close friends about emotions. Expressing feelings of frustration will help Jen and other people to better understand the internal distress.

WORK
Approach volunteer groups for work that may be more suited to current abilities and lifestyle.

EMOTIONAL HEALTH
Address problems with self-esteem by talking to a therapist about the issues that are causing constant anxiety and frustration.

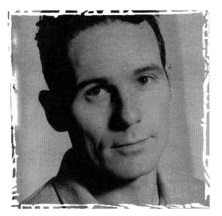

EMOTIONAL HEALTH
Physical and psychological setbacks can undermine self-esteem and mental well-being.

FAMILY
Emotional responsibility for a family can often be more demanding than financial obligations.

WORK
Work is a major source of interaction and independence. Not being able to find suitable employment can be stressful.

HOW THINGS TURNED OUT FOR STEVE

Steve went to see a cognitive therapist, who discussed his self-perception with him. The therapist helped Steve to recognize how he was selectively focusing on the negative aspects of his life, magnifying them to the point where he lost sight of the good things. Steve learned to refute some of his negative feelings and reaffirm the positive, which enabled him to take pleasure in his friends and family once again and accept their support.

SEASONAL AFFECTIVE DISORDER

For some people repeated episodes of depression are as predictable as the changing seasons. Usually with the arrival of winter, sufferers experience a deterioration in their energy levels, enthusiasm, and general mental health.

Scientists believe that the disorder is caused by a decrease in the amount of sunlight to which these individuals are exposed. One explanation is that darkness enhances the production of melatonin, a natural chemical secreted by the pineal gland that has a sedative effect on the body, thus increasing fatigue and reducing physical activity. With extra melatonin, lethargy and depression can occur more frequently during the winter months.

From all the extensive research that has been conducted over many years, the conclusion is that most mood disorders result from several interacting factors. The majority of therapists now believe that clinical depression is nearly always caused by some combination of biological and social factors. The biological angle is supported by the fact that if one identical twin becomes clinically depressed, there is a 67 percent chance that the other will also experience a mental disorder at some point in life. Although this indicates a distinct genetic connection, the 33 percent who are not affected suggests that biology cannot be the only factor. Sociocultural factors must also play a role in determining a person's susceptibility.

Even though some people are biologically predisposed to depression, the fact remains that many of them never actually suffer from the problem. Some of the research in this area suggests that this is because these individuals never encounter any trigger events that could bring on the condition. People with stable homes and relationships and lifelong support from family and friends seem to be less likely to develop depression.

A study conducted in London in the 1970s found that women suffering from depression tended to have few friends and were socially isolated. These individuals had also experienced more stressful events in the preceding 12 months than women who were not depressed. These results appear to indicate that a combination of recent life events and personal tendencies can greatly affect an individual's susceptibility to depression.

The role of nutrition and drugs

Chemical imbalances in the body, possibly brought on by insufficient amounts of certain nutrients or by medications, can also contribute to the onset of depression. Some nutrients that have been implicated in depression include most of the B vitamins, folic acid, vitamin C, and omega-3 fatty acids. Depressed people tend to have lower than normal lipid levels of these nutrients.

Medications for which depression is often a side effect include beta blockers for hypertension, digoxin and other drugs for heart disease, some antihistamines, oral contraceptives and other hormones, some

continued on page 104

ARE WOMEN MORE VULNERABLE TO DEPRESSION THAN MEN?

Research suggests that women are almost twice as likely as men to experience depression, although scientists have no clear answers as to why. Some believe that hormones play a significant role, while others claim that the condition is caused by X-chromosome abnormalities and, because women have two X chromosomes, they are more prone to the illness. Still others believe that Western society makes impossibly high and conflicting demands on women, which lead to higher levels of guilt and lower self-esteem. It could be, however, that women are no more prone to depression than men but that doctors tend to reach this particular diagnosis with female patients. While women are more inclined to admit their depression and seek professional help, statistics reveal that men turn more often to alcohol or other self-medication and perhaps are not diagnosed as often.

The Psychiatric Team

A person suffering from some kind of mental disorder may see a psychiatrist or other therapist for help, and this person may be backed up by a team of different specialists, each of whom will contribute to the patient's therapy.

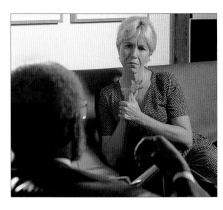

CONSULTING A THERAPIST
The first stage of any psychiatric treatment involves sitting down and discussing your problems with a mental health professional.

THE PSYCHIATRIC TEAM
A patient and his wife (top) are sitting down with a psychiatric team—psychiatrist, psychiatric nurse, social worker, and occupational therapist—to discuss the different stages and aspects that his treatment will involve.

Receiving psychiatric treatment can involve one professional or a team of different consultants, depending on the complexity of the problem. A team has the advantage of offering a variety of services, all of them coordinated to meet the special needs of the patient. For example, a person with schizophrenia will need the help of not only a psychiatrist, who will prescribe medication and provide psychotherapy, but also a psychiatric nurse, who is qualified to monitor and assist with medications, an occupational therapist, who can help with learning new skills or relearning old ones, and a social worker, who can be instrumental in helping the patient become reintegrated into the community after a hospital stay.

Sometimes formal meetings are arranged in order to discuss the care program. The whole team will be present at such meetings and will provide advice on everything from medication to Social Security benefits. It is important that a patient's partner or primary caregiver be included in

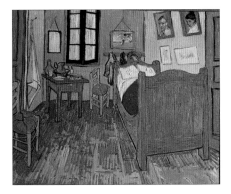

PSYCHOLOGY TEST
Clients are sometimes asked to relate the feelings they experience when looking at photographic images or works of art, such as this painting by Van Gogh, Bedroom at Arles.

discussions and offered practical help and advice. Many times all those who are concerned with the problem will be invited to sit down together and discuss the condition and its treatment.

The psychiatrist will usually lead the discussion and advise the patient about medication and its potential side effects. After the initial assessments and therapy sessions, the psychiatrist will probably see the patient only periodically in order to establish whether treatment is going according to plan. The psychiatrist will be given regular updates, however, by the psychiatric nurse on the case, who will monitor the patient regularly, perhaps visiting the client at home, providing support, and checking that there are no unexpected side effects from the medication. Sometimes a clinical psychologist will be asked to provide psychological assessment and therapy as well.

An occupational therapist is sometimes involved to provide advice on the practical problems of living with a mental disorder. Both patient and primary caregiver will have to be advised on the likely difficulties they will encounter, such as any increasing debilitating effects, and told about the facilities that are available to help improve the quality of life. Maintaining independent living while suffering from a severe

mental disorder can be extremely difficult, and both the sufferer and the family will need emotional support.

A social worker attends care program meetings in order to provide advice about financial arrangements and community services. Providing guidance on benefits and resources, the social worker will help with the practical problems of living with a psychological disorder.

How do mental health professionals assess a problem?

In order to assess the problems and needs of a patient, a psychiatrist will interview him or her. This can range from a small informal chat to a highly organized battery of tests. During a clinical interview, the psychiatrist will question the patient about symptoms and background history. The patient's behavior and mood will also be observed because this can provide clues to the nature of the problem. These meetings are generally a good way to establish rapport with the patient so that further, more intense analyses will seem less threatening.

Are practical tests used in making an analysis?

Sometimes a mental health professional, usually a clinical psychologist, will use practical tests, or questionnaires, as part of a patient's assessment. To develop such questionnaires, a set of questions has been asked of a number of people at different times and the responses have been collected and analyzed to provide statistical norms. The test is then given to a person who is thought to need psychological help, and that person's responses are compared with those from the statistical norm in order to establish how unusual the patient's emotional responses and behavior actually are.

Personality inventories, in which subjects are asked to indicate how typical or out of the ordinary a series of statements about themselves are, can be one useful way of monitoring

self-perception. If a client tends to answer questions in the same way as people in a certain diagnostic group, this will help categorize the problem.

Projective personality tests may also be used. These are designed to encourage a patient to give automatic responses to certain colors or images. The figures or objects that the patient reports seeing will help the professional to analyze some of the different influences that are affecting the patient.

Paintings are a particularly good way to encourage a client to project his or her feelings onto another object. By discussing the feelings that an image evokes, the patient may reveal a certain level of disturbance.

Intelligence tests may be used as well to ascertain if there are any cognitive problems. All of the above tests, however, are inconclusive without further analysis. A psychiatrist needs to build up a picture of the problem, and this involves comprehensive analysis and discussion, all of which take fully into account the patient's feelings and symptoms.

WHAT YOU CAN DO AT HOME

It would, of course, be very unwise to attempt any unsupervised self-treatment for a psychological disorder. You can help yourself, however, by becoming aware of symptoms and acknowledging that you have a problem if one is indicated. It is important to be emotionally open with yourself and accept that irrational thoughts, extended bouts of sadness, and such physical symptoms as long-term chronic pain could be indications of a need for therapy.

Recognizing a mental problem and coming to terms with inner conflicts at an early stage can help prevent a disorder from becoming severe. And a good therapist can guide you in realizing and addressing your problems in your own time.

painkillers, and corticosteroids. People who suffer from such serious diseases as cancer are also more prone to depression, but it is not certain whether the illness causes a change in brain chemistry or they are simply depressed from wrestling with it.

The role of brain mechanisms

The brain is made up of billions of neurons, nerve cells that communicate with each other through chemical messengers called neurotransmitters. The neurotransmitters flow across the synaptic gap between each neuron, and it is variations in their activity that scientists believe are implicated in depression. There are many different types of neurotransmitters, but the two that are most important in relation to depression are noradrenaline and serotonin. Depressed persons tend to have lower than normal levels.

The type of message and neurotransmitter combine to affect a person's behavior. For example, if a message that will potentially cause a positive reaction in a person is met by high levels of serotonin, the result can be strong response emotions and activity. If it is met by low serotonin levels, the message may fail to be transmitted efficiently, and little or no response will occur. For this reason a depressed person may find it difficult to interpret positive events as a potential mood booster. Antidepressants are often prescribed to alleviate symptoms by raising levels of the appropriate neurotransmitters.

Cognitive therapy for depression

There are several therapeutic approaches used for treating unipolar depression, but cognitive therapy has proven particularly useful in dealing with the serious bouts of misery and self-hatred that occur with most cases. Cognitive therapy works by identify-

DRUGS

A number of drugs are available for treating depression, although these can only help relieve symptoms and do not address the cause. Unipolar depression is often treated with MAO (monoamine oxidase) inhibitors and tricyclics, which increase the concentration of neurotransmitters like serotonin in the synaptic gap. Antidepressants can take a while to become effective, however, and so psychotherapies are often used alongside treatment with medications.

Bipolar depression is more complex to treat because the patient needs to be stabilized between two manic states. Lithium is useful in regulating neurotransmission and creating a balance between the two bipolar states. It works on a principle similar to that of insulin for diabetics, reducing the effect of manic swings and helping to maintain stability. Nevertheless, researchers are still trying to find a more specific treatment for this condition.

ing and testing the patient's assumptions, beliefs, and ways of thinking and teaching him or her skills for dealing with depression. By addressing low self-esteem, for example, cognitive therapy can help the patient work toward understanding the reasons behind a depressed mood. If the person claims to be a failure, for example, the therapist will encourage him or her to evaluate the validity of the statement. By pointing out that the patient has had successful experiences and that events do not always turn out negatively, the therapist aids in refuting the original opinion and improving the client's self-esteem.

As patients increase the number of their positive activities, they learn to monitor and counter automatic negative thoughts. By gaining this control, they become empowered to alter moods. Although more expensive than most drug treatment, cognitive therapy is often more effective at preventing relapses. (Chapter 6 looks at other types of therapy that address thought patterns.)

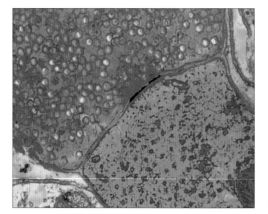

NERVE TRANSMISSION
This electron micrograph shows how messages are transmitted from one neuron, or nerve cell (pink), to another (blue). As the message impulse reaches the end of the neuron, neurotransmitters diffuse it across the tiny synaptic gap, and it binds with receptors on the other side.

THE BIOLOGY OF DEPRESSION

Scientists believe that depression may be at least partly caused by the levels of certain neurotransmitters in the brain. The chemical serotonin helps to transmit emotional messages, such as happiness, love, and anger. If there are insufficient supplies of serotonin, impulses will not be passed efficiently from one neuron to the next, and the person will not experience the appropriate mood enhancement.

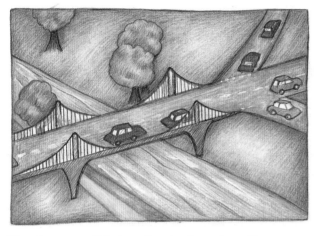

When there are sufficient supplies of such neurotransmitters as serotonin, emotional impulses can cross the synaptic gap between neurons and pass along appropriate messages to elevate mood.

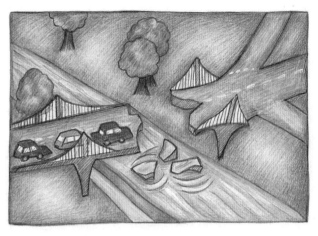

If the mood-elevating message is unable to cross the synaptic gap for lack of the appropriate neurotransmitter, the good feeling will not be conveyed, and the person will remain in a depressed state.

MANIC DEPRESSION

Manic, or bipolar, depression is much less common than unipolar depression, but it is a debilitating disease, typically characterized by both energetic elation and extreme despair. Patients may occasionally suffer from both ends of the emotional spectrum simultaneously, but it is more usual to alternate between the two states, with each one lasting for days, weeks, or even months.

During the manic phase, individuals may exhibit a range of symptoms, including hyperactivity, exaggerated optimism and self-importance, recklessness, extravagance, and racing speech and flow of ideas. These symptoms are offset by the fatigue, low self-esteem, pessimism, anxiety, and chronic sadness usually experienced during the depressive phase. Although the energetic optimism of the manic stage may seem an appealing contrast to lethargic depression, these feelings are largely superficial and desperate, masking a disturbed state of mind.

The roller-coaster effect can be severely disruptive, and friends, colleagues, and family members are often unsure about how to deal with each situation. It would be fair to say that the manic episodes of the bipolar depressive complicate, rather than alleviate, the sadness in their lives.

The biology of manic depression

Unlike unipolar depression, for which biological, psychoanalytical, cognitive, and social theories still compete, manic depression is largely attributed to biology. While chronic depression appears to be partly caused by low levels of noradrenaline, the manic state of bipolar disorders is generally associated with excessive quantities of the chemical. It seems that sufferers tend to have consistently high levels of this important neurotransmitter in the nervous system, which would confirm that they have a genetic predisposition to the illness.

Close relatives of manic depressives have about a one in five chance of also developing the disease. For those who do not have a close relative who is bipolar, the chance of being affected is reduced to 1 in 100. Interestingly, there are no sex differences in the rate at which bipolar depression occurs, although once a person has developed the illness, it is likely to recur for a considerable period of time. Stress, in particular, can be a trigger for further relapses, as can discontinuation of medication or treatment. Because of its biological foundation, the main form of treatment is the drug lithium, although research is being conducted into other potential treatments and therapies.

ANXIETY DISORDERS AND PHOBIAS

Everybody experiences anxiety at some point in their life. If these feelings are intense or persist for long periods of time, however, they can become harmful and debilitating.

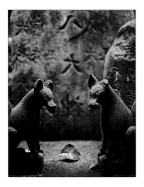

LOCAL DEPRESSION
Some disorders are culture specific. In a few isolated areas of Japan, for example, foxes have a mythological aura, causing some people to suffer from a condition known as kitsunetsuki – *a fear of being possessed by foxes. This condition is virtually unknown anywhere else in the world.*

It is perfectly normal to respond to the various pressures and events of the world around us with some anxiety. We all worry about tests or job interviews or become tense in threatening or unfamiliar situations. In some people, however, these feelings can turn into panic that inhibits normal life, possibly even affecting their ability to work or socialize. It is estimated that these emotional disorders affect about 15 percent of the population at any one time in the form of anxiety or panic attacks or phobias. Most of us know somebody who reacts to certain situations in this way. When a person exhibits a morbid fear of spiders or of travel in an airplane, he or she reveals how we can all be subject to irrational behavior, dismissing logical thought in our attempt to avoid unwelcome confrontation with our fears.

ANXIETY DISORDERS

Anxiety occurs when the mind perceives a discrepancy between an event facing us and our ability to cope with it. The nervous system responds by raising blood pressure and heartbeat and supplying extra oxygen to the brain as it analyzes the conflicting information. An anxiety disorder is distinguished from everyday anxiety by three factors: it is

---

PROCESSING ANXIETY

People who suffer from anxiety disorders tend to have distorted views of the world and perceive things out of all proportion or context. One theory concerning such behavior is that anxious people often seek out or notice more readily any information that relates to their anxieties. In an investigation conducted in 1993, scientists found that sufferers of anxiety are actually more sensitive to disturbing stimuli, often tuning in to them before the information has entered conscious awareness. The subjects were asked to name the colors of patches while ignoring the anxiety-related words written on them. With extremely brief exposure to the words, participants rarely had time to read the phrases, but the colors that they could recall all had negative words, like *embarrassed*, on them. This shows how sufferers of anxiety disorders direct more attention to processing information that relates to their inhibitions and fears.

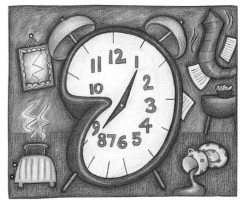

ANXIETY REINFORCEMENT
People who suffer from an anxiety disorder tend to focus on things that reinforce their fears, such as the problem of time when running late for work or an interview.

WHAT CAUSES PANIC DISORDERS?

Both biological and psychological factors are involved in panic disorders. Some studies have shown that panic disorders tend to run in families, suggesting that genetics may play a significant role in vulnerability. Other studies have shown that people with panic disorders are overtly sensitive to physical arousal. For example, someone who suffers from a panic disorder may react to a stimulant like caffeine with a panic attack, whereas a nonsufferer would simply find it a useful pick-me-up. Cognitive therapists try to get sufferers of panic attacks to reinterpret the physical signs of arousal as nonthreatening. For instance, when a patient's heart starts to pound, he or she is encouraged to stop interpreting this as catastrophic and frightening.

irrational, uncontrollable, and disruptive. Irrationality stems from the fact that the perceived threat is exaggerated and the individual is responding disproportionately to it. The anxiety is uncontrollable because the person feels unable to stop it, no matter how inappropriate the response is. The response is disruptive because it interferes with relationships, work, and everyday activities.

People who suffer from a free-floating anxiety disorder do not usually have a specific focus for their distress. This anxiety is a pervasive sensation that causes restlessness, poor sleep, and general discomfort. Panic attacks, on the other hand, have all the symptoms of general anxiety but are often linked to a specific situation. The symptoms may then develop into a phobia as the individual increasingly dreads confronting a situation that might bring on an attack. Fainting in an anxious situation, for example, might lead to agoraphobia (fear of open space), with the person dreading the prospect of losing control and experiencing a panic attack in a public place. Many patients will go to great lengths to avoid what they believe triggers their attacks. Refusing to fly and avoiding hospitals are two examples of how personal fears and anxieties can affect the way a person lives.

PHOBIAS

Phobias are excessive and irrational fears of specific objects or situations that have a disruptive effect on an individual's normal functioning. Many people suffer from terrors of this kind, ranging from an extreme response to certain animals or situations to fear of injections or treatment by a dentist.

Heights or enclosed spaces often bring on trepidation because an individual is forced to deal with a situation that is unfamiliar or greatly different from that of normal daily life. There are many phobias, however, that reveal anxiety about something not generally regarded as threatening. Such phobias as fear of empty rooms (kenophobia), beards (pogonophobia), even snow (chionophobia) have all been recognized as real, although uncommon conditions.

One distinguishing feature of phobias is that they foster irrational behavior. While many people become anxious when encountering a new social situation, for instance, a phobic person will allow this fear to prevent interaction with others. This behavior will inevitably inhibit social development. A phobic person might also see several different situations as equally threatening. The difference between public speaking and attending an informal gathering is vast, but both situations can seem equally daunting to an individual who associates them both with needing to fulfill an impossible role. Extreme self-consciousness and a belief that all interaction must be measured can lead a person to avoid all social occasions.

How do phobias develop?

Phobias are generally acquired through learning and conditioning, particularly during childhood. A frightening confrontation with a dog at a young age, for example,

DID YOU KNOW?
Phobias are often brought on by a bad experience. Because we learn to avoid painful stimulants, phobias related to wasps, snakes, or falling from a high place are more common than phobias related to trees or gerbils. The common fear of spiders may derive from genetic programming from our ancestors, although living in the wild exposed us to more dangerous creatures than the common household creepy-crawly.

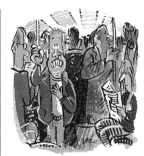

CLAUSTROPHOBIA
Fear of enclosed spaces with no easy exit can lead people to avoid using elevators or trains.

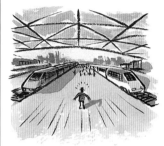

AGORAPHOBIA
Fear of open space, as opposed to the security of home, can make going out a daunting experience.

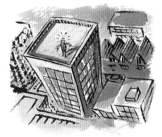

ACROPHOBIA
An irrational fear of heights has been known to prevent people from ascending tall buildings.

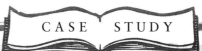

A Social Phobic

Social phobics are people who fear being judged and evaluated by other people. They embarrass easily and may experience great self-consciousness when being introduced to strangers, especially people in authority. Most become very distressed and nervous when they are the center of attention or have to say something in a public situation.

Susan, 23 years old, graduated from college with honors and has recently started work in a responsible job at the national headquarters of a leading charitable organization. Susan has always been nervous about standing out at social events, and at college she hated being asked to lead a debate or present her work. Now she finds that she must give presentations to senior managers and outside groups, and this part of her job terrifies her. Building up to and during a presentation, she experiences intense palpitations, sweating, and even some breathing difficulties, and she feels she has made a complete mess of every presentation. She is worried that she appears incompetent to her superiors and not up to the job.

WHAT SHOULD SUSAN DO?

Susan should acknowledge that she has a social phobia and that this is a challenge in her life that she can and will overcome. Although many people have some fear of public speaking, she needs to recognize that her fears are extreme and irrational.

Consulting a therapist may help her come to terms with her problem. Susan could benefit from the help of a cognitive therapist, who will encourage her gradually to confront the social and work situations that she dreads. By practicing her presentation skills on a group of close friends or working on her anxieties with other people who have similar problems, Susan can acquire the confidence to believe in her own performance.

Action Plan

WORK
Practice presentations on friends or family members and work with a therapist to build confidence.

STRESS
Learn deep-breathing techniques to help manage moments of work-related stress. Keep unnecessary stress factors, such as being rushed, to a minimum before social events.

EMOTIONAL HEALTH
Prepare a step-by-step plan of action that will make you feel more relaxed and psychologically prepared for presentations.

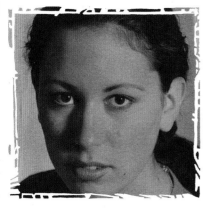

EMOTIONAL HEALTH
Anxiety can breed further stress and lead to emotional and physical health problems.

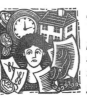

WORK
Presentations, increasingly common in all professional roles, can produce great anxiety.

STRESS
When the external factors that cause stress are dealt with, the pressure can be greatly reduced.

HOW THINGS TURNED OUT FOR SUSAN

Susan saw a therapist who helped her first to understand some of her irrational fears and then to find ways of coping with them. The therapist also recommended she join a toast-master's or discussion group to help improve her ability to speak on a range of subjects.

Susan took training in presentation skills and learned how to prepare material impeccably. This has greatly improved her confidence in her performance and effectiveness.

FEAR OF FLYING

Air travel is something that most people take for granted, but for others a fear of flying can cause a great deal of distress and disruption in life. Like most other phobias, however, the fear of flying can be treated with specific counseling sessions. Many airlines have developed courses that teach nervous passengers how to manage and eventually overcome their fear. Open to anyone, the courses usually run for a day, involve discussions about the flight process, and simulate some of the noises and movements that a plane makes.

Specially trained psychologists also explore with the group various aspects of their fear, such as what might be causing it, and teach relaxation techniques to help passengers avoid panic responses while on a flight. The day may culminate with an hour's flight with both the crew and the therapists.

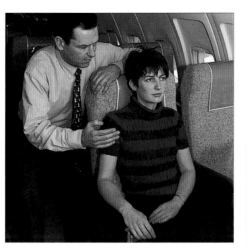

IN THE PLANE
Some airlines offer a program that includes taking people up in a plane and giving one-on-one coaching in relaxation methods. Therapists talk them through a flight and offer help during difficult moments, encouraging participants to assess the principal causes of their fear.

could lead to a person avoiding dogs for years to come. By keeping away from the anxiety triggers, the individual never learns to manage the fear, and so the phobia is never cured. The response, moreover, may become so generalized that all animals of a similar nature are avoided.

Some people may acquire a phobia by observing the fearful reactions of someone else. It is common for children to develop the same fears that their parents have, through observing and imitating the behavior of their role models.

Therapies to combat phobias

Because therapists generally believe that phobias are developed through learning and behavior, most of them work to retrain an individual's thought patterns. By gradually confronting the patient with benign aspects of the offending trigger, the therapist encourages the individual to recognize the irrationality of his or her behavior and learn to adjust the responses accordingly.

Cognitive behavior therapy works by helping the patient to realize that the trigger is actually harmless. A fear of horses, for example, might first be addressed by encouraging the sufferer to study and come to terms with a photograph of the animal.

Then the sound of a horse might be introduced and other specific features that increasingly involve the fearful person with the animal. More advanced levels might involve looking at real horses in controlled circumstances until the person can touch a horse without supervision. The psychologist helps the person progressively deal with each level, all the time maintaining a sense of calmness until the fear is conquered.

Recent research has been conducted into taking some of these assimilations one step further. Dr. Larry Hodges and Dr. Barbara Rothbaum of the Georgia Institute of Technology have been experimenting with virtual reality computing as an aid to treating such conditions as acrophobia (fear of heights). In order to confront greater degrees of height, the patient sits in a computer laboratory wearing virtual reality headsets. An experience similar to that of the perception and movement of depth in a high place is then transmitted through the visor. This helps clients to become accustomed to heights while secure on the ground.

VIRTUAL REALITY
Therapies that encourage sufferers to encounter stimulants similar to those that cause their phobia are becoming increasingly popular. For people who fear heights, virtual reality can simulate many of the same sensations that are encountered in high places while the subject remains safe on the ground.

ADDICTION

Every day millions of people take substances that alter how they feel. While many of these chemicals are legal and may even have been prescribed, they should always be used with care.

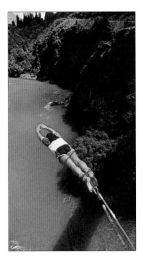

ACTIVITY ADDICTION
Anything that affects the mind and body has the potential to become addictive. Some people become addicted to sports like bungee jumping, which bring on an intense adrenaline rush.

All drugs and other chemicals that affect the way the body or mind functions can be dangerous if misused. Although some are more dangerous than others, it is always best to avoid regular use of any stimulant or other chemical that provides pleasure or support for sagging moods. If your mind and body become too accustomed to or dependent on them, you may lose the ability to function fully and efficiently without them. Certain activities can also become addictive.

CAUSES OF ADDICTION

There are two types of addiction: physiological and psychological. Physiological addictions involve substances that the body comes to depend on for normal functioning, whereas psychological dependencies are more often related to activities—gambling, surfing the Internet, and bungee jumping, for example. Such activities may provide both a biological adrenaline rush and an emotional buzz that can become difficult to give up. Certain drugs—alcohol and cocaine, for instance—are also addictive both physiologically and psychologically.

In the case of substance, or chemical, addiction, as the body adapts to the active elements in the substance and incorporates them as part of normal functioning, it builds up a certain level of tolerance. This forces the user to increase the amount of the substance progressively in order to maintain the same level of pleasure. If the chemical is subsequently not taken, the body will be unable

---

THE ADDICTION CYCLE

Addictions work by making either the mind or body reliant on a particular stimulant. As we become used to physically and mentally functioning with the presence of a stimulant, we eventually become dependent on it, and gradually more and more of the stimulant is needed to sustain normal bodily and mental functioning. The motive for taking a stimulant in the first place is to experience its sensations. But as the body and mind become adjusted to working normally with the chemical, the individual needs to take increasing amounts simply to continue feeling the stimulant's effects. Needing to increase your consumption of a stimulant just to sustain a normal effect or feeling that you cannot function without shows that you have become mentally and physically dependent on it. This cycle applies to both drugs and activities.

DOWNWARD SPIRAL
What begins as the occasional use of a stimulant can lead to a downward spiral of addiction as the mind and body learn to rely on regular, increasingly large doses.

to work properly and may suffer from withdrawal. The buildup of tolerance to a drug can be relatively slow, as with alcohol, or rapid, as in the case of heroin.

With psychological dependence, the body learns to sustain normal functioning while under the influence of a particular chemical or activity. As tolerance builds up, further psychological adjustments are made, and the mind comes to depend increasingly on the stimulating, exciting, or feel-good effect of the activity or substance. Larger doses are then needed to achieve the same level of pleasure. Eventually emotional relationships, self-esteem, normal social behavior, even outward identity can seem impossible or dreary to maintain without the addictive stimulation. As with physiological dependence, withdrawal symptoms may occur if the stimulant is removed. This is because the mind becomes adapted to and dependent on the sensations that these chemicals or activities provide just as the body does.

TYPES OF SUBSTANCE ADDICTION

There are a number of chemicals that can become addictive for the user. Many are part of everyday products and affect the mind and body in mild ways. Others can be so potent that addiction happens quickly and is very difficult to overcome.

Tranquilizers and painkillers

Tranquilizers, including anxiolytic (anxiety-reducing) drugs like Valium and Librium, are commonly prescribed for people with nervous disorders. They help relieve anxiety by increasing production of the neurotransmitter gamma-amino-butyric acid (GABA), which inhibits activity in the part of the brain that controls emotion. Doctors monitor usage carefully. Although the potential damage of tranquilizer dependence is less than that of many other prescription drugs, if the body and mind are allowed to become too dependent on these chemicals, they will lose the ability to maintain normal levels of relaxation.

Barbiturates, which work by depressing the nervous system and reducing mental alertness, are now rarely used for treating anxiety, but they are sometimes contained in sleeping pills. High doses can cause wide swings of emotion. Large quantities can also lead to slow muscle response and potential respiratory failure, so dependence is more

TYPES OF DRUGS

Different types of drugs affect the body in various ways. Drugs that alter the consciousness in some manner generally fall into one of the categories that are described below:

TYPE OF DRUG	EFFECTS ON THE BODY
Depressants	Depressants reduce the activity of the nervous system and dull the senses to such forms of discomfort as pain and cold. Alcohol is the most commonly used depressant, but barbiturates, found in some sleeping pills and relaxants, also reduce mental and physiological activity.
Stimulants	As their name suggests, stimulants produce feelings of energy and motivation. Amphetamines and cocaine are two powerful stimulants that raise blood pressure and yield short periods of pleasurable sensations. When the effects wear off, however, the user often experiences a sudden letdown, with profound fatigue, anxiety, and depression.
Opiates	Extremely dangerous drugs, opiates, such as morphine, heroin, and opium, produce a feeling of lethargy and a marked slowing down of virtually all bodily functions. They also affect consciousness and often induce a dreamlike state. Prolonged use can inhibit the body's ability to deal with pain and can lead to addiction and the need for increasing quantities of the drug.
Psychedelics and hallucinogens	Psychedelics, such as marijuana, alter sensory perceptions, and hallucinogens, such as LSD, generate sensory perceptions without external stimuli. Both drug types affect an individual's ability to judge his or her surroundings correctly. While marijuana is associated with relaxation, LSD can cause a variety of extreme sensations, including elation, fear, insecurity, and depression.

dangerous than an addiction to anxiolytic substances. Other types of painkillers, like morphine—often referred to as opiates because of their opium-like effect on the brain—vary in their addictive potential and damaging side effects.

Hard drugs

Like morphine, the illegal drug heroin is an opiate and effectively reduces physiological and mental activity. However, it is much more dangerous because developing tolerance to it and a subsequent addiction is often very rapid. There are also dangers from infected needles and impure mixtures of the drug, which are further intensified by the difficulty of calculating the amount needed to obtain a pleasurable high. Addicts can easily take an unintentional overdose, with life-threatening consequences.

Withdrawal symptoms from heroin occur almost immediately, and addicts display physiological and psychological distress as soon as a "fix" has worn off. The symptoms get progressively worse for up to 72 hours

The high price of drugs

Many famous movie stars and other personalities have fallen victim to some kind of drug dependency. The Welsh poet Dylan Thomas died of alcohol poisoning at only 39, and the French singer Edith Piaf was notorious for her addictions to alcohol and morphine. However, there are also examples of famous people who have overcome their addictions and continued to pursue successful careers.

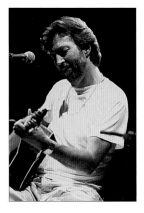

DEFEATING ADDICTION
Rock star Eric Clapton successfully overcame an addiction to cocaine.

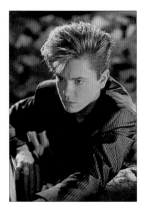

SUCCUMBING TO THE DANGER
River Phoenix was a young movie star who died tragically as a result of drug abuse.

NATURAL STIMULANTS

Although people often turn to chemicals to stimulate the mind and body, there are many natural ways to achieve a calmer or more energized state without the risk of serious side effects or potential damage.

▶ *Many herbal teas provide a healthful and natural way to stimulate or relax the mind. Peppermint, lemon zest, and ginger can all be energizing; chamomile and valerian teas help promote a calm and relaxed state.*

▶ *Yoga, massage, and meditation can all relax the body and clear the mind. Aromatherapy with bath oils or candles can also help to induce a state of peace and tranquillity.*

▶ *Physical exercise increases the brain's production of endorphins, which contribute to a natural high.*

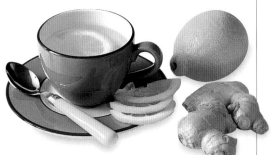

HERBAL INFUSIONS
Many herbal drinks can help to relax or stimulate the body and are generally safer than other, potentially addictive chemicals.

and then eventually subside, usually disappearing after about a week. Psychological dependency, however, can continue for many years or even a lifetime.

Alcohol

Alcohol lowers tension and anxiety by depressing the nervous system and reducing social inhibition. Common abuse of the drug has led to the highest social cost of all drug addictions. Alcohol affects judgment and impairs motor skills—even in small amounts—but its long-term health effects are especially damaging. Alcohol is related to a high percentage of automobile accidents, birth defects, liver and heart conditions, and brain damage. It also adversely affects numerous other conditions that are not specifically related to alcohol.

It is estimated that two-thirds of the adult population in North America drink alcohol at least occasionally and up to 20 percent of these people will go through a period of dependency at some point in their lives. The consequences can be damaging—mentally, physically, and financially. One key factor in overcoming an addiction is to admit that a problem exists. Many people dependent on alcohol continue to insist that the situation is within their control. Once they have accepted that they need help, however, there are numerous support groups, such as Alcoholics Anonymous, that can provide encouragement and assistance.

Caffeine

Caffeine is a stimulant that raises levels of serotonin, dopamine, and noradrenaline in the brain. It is found in coffee but is also present (at about one-third of the strength in coffee) in cola drinks and in tea. Its overall effect is to increase alertness, although excessive quantities can lead to nervousness and increased heart rate. It has been found that people who habitually drink two or more cups a day can suffer from withdrawal symptoms, especially headaches, if they stop their caffeine intake suddenly.

Smoking

Nicotine is one of the most widely used addictive stimulants. It is commonly taken by smoking tobacco and presents numerous health risks, such as lung cancer and cardiovascular disease. Even so, people continue to smoke, claiming that a cigarette helps to calm their nerves and relax them. In fact, small doses of nicotine actually increase mental alertness and speed up bodily functioning. Nicotine reduces fatigue and stimulates heartbeat, so only large doses have the potential to act as a depressant.

When a cigarette is inhaled, nicotine reaches the brain in seconds, but its effect lasts for only about 30 minutes. Chain smokers generally feel the need to maintain steady nicotine levels, and thus they smoke a cigarette about every half hour or so. Dependency on nicotine builds up very quickly—much more rapidly than with alcohol—and many people become very reliant on its properties. It can be extremely addictive, both physiologically and psychologically, so withdrawal symptoms are common as the body attempts to return to a normal functioning state.

COMBATING ADDICTION

Different types of addiction require different kinds of therapy, and the physiological, psychological, social, and even legal consequences of a dependency often call for multiple layers of treatment and support. In most cases the treatment strategy for an addiction includes gradual withdrawal from the substance, whether this means forsaking morning coffee or receiving supervised help in overcoming a drug addiction. With serious addictions, psychological therapy is also needed as a rule to help an individual gain confidence in his or her ability to function without the addictive substance. This approach generally improves self-esteem and helps reduce the risk of a relapse.

Many addictions can never be entirely overcome but simply kept at bay with ongoing support. Alcoholics, for example, are usually taught to be constantly aware of their problem, never believing that it is safe to return to controlled or even occasional drinking. Ongoing support from "buddies" and self-help groups aims to provide a framework and atmosphere for addicts to pursue ongoing recovery. Similarly, some residential communities for drug-related addictions use a combination of specially trained therapists and fellow sufferers to help an addict pull through the difficult time of rehabilitation. Essentially, however, an individual can hope to overcome an addiction only if he or she has sufficient will and belief in self. Therapists are now increasingly encouraging the practice of yoga and various types of meditation to help addicts find inner strength and commitment.

Relapsing

With all addictions, a relapse can be a major problem, and both families of addicts and professionals must be able to recognize potential danger points. If recovery is slow or if the original lifestyle or source of discontent that caused addiction returns, the recovering addict may well relapse. As with any treatment, the emotional and psychological causes of a problem need to be addressed for a person to recover fully.

Addiction substitution

When one addiction is being conquered, there is always a risk that the addicted person will become dependent on another substance or habit to fulfill his or her psychological or physiological needs. Evidence suggests that many addictive substances, such as nicotine, alcohol, heroin, and antidepressants, increase levels of the neurotransmitter dopamine, which is associated with sensations of pleasure. A drop or deficiency in this natural chemical may cause an individual to seek other substances that enhance its production.

SELF-HELP IN OVERCOMING ADDICTION

Some addictions can best be overcome with the help of professionals, but there are things you can do yourself to break a habit or aid in your therapy. One is meditation. Many recovering drug abusers have used transcendental meditation to help them overcome their addiction. The procedure is to stretch the body into a relaxed state and then repeat a word or set of words known as a mantra. This helps focus the mind and reduce inner tension.

STRETCH FIRST
Before beginning your meditation, stretch every muscle consecutively to promote bodily relaxation.

▶ *Find a quiet, peaceful location and choose an appropriate mantra that is easy to remember and meaningful to you.*

▶ *Silently repeat your mantra over and over again, focusing your attention on it and not allowing your concentration to slip. This does take practice, but self-discipline and commitment will greatly help.*

▶ *Continue the meditation session for 15 to 20 minutes. Practice meditating several times a week, particularly when you feel under stress or are tempted to resort to your addiction.*

A Compulsive Gambler

Behavioral addictions can be as mentally and socially destructive as substance dependencies. Because the addiction is not always physically evident, individuals can for a time hide their symptoms from family, friends, and even themselves. This increases the destructive effects of the addiction as the person becomes increasingly involved in deceit and self-delusion.

Mike is a 27-year-old car salesman who is engaged to Sandra. He is intelligent and successful in a challenging job in executive car sales. For the past six months, however, Mike has been gambling heavily. Following a hot tip from an acquaintance, Mike had a big win and a tremendous thrill. Now he finds himself betting on a whole range of sports and other activities, often staying up until four or five in the morning to monitor races and competitions.

Although Sandra has tried to stop him from gambling, she has no idea how serious his addiction is or how much debt he has gotten into. He insists he can stop whenever he wants to but is just waiting for another big win before he does.

WHAT SHOULD MIKE DO?

Mike must admit that he has a problem and do it soon. He needs to learn how to readjust his psychological systems so that they do not depend on gambling. If he can live without gambling for six months, his mind will be on its way to readjusting itself to normal life, but he must be prepared to apply discipline and self-control.

Mike will need the unquestioning and uncritical support of his partner and the practical support of his employer, but he should also consider attending a therapy group or Gamblers Anonymous. With the empathetic understanding of other addicts, he should be able to find the determination and faith that he needs to overcome his addiction.

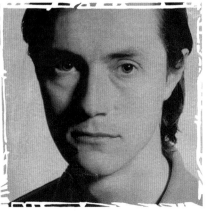

EMOTIONAL HEALTH
Fooling yourself about your self-control can be emotionally dangerous.

PARTNER/SPOUSE
The partners of addicted gamblers suffer in many ways—physically, financially, and emotionally.

FINANCES
Gamblers beg, steal, and borrow to raise funds. This not only leads to financial difficulties but also saps the strength and sympathy of those who are trying to help them.

Action Plan

PARTNER/SPOUSE
Admit to partner the full extent of the problem and ask for support in dealing with it. Be honest in order to maintain a sense of trust.

FINANCES
Stop gambling expenditures entirely; don't attempt to just reduce them. Debt counseling can be helpful in organizing repayments and dealing with creditors.

EMOTIONAL HEALTH
Find a support group for sharing experiences and learning coping strategies.

HOW THINGS TURNED OUT FOR MIKE

After two years, a lot of heartache, and help from a therapy group that specializes in gambling, Mike has finally broken free of his addiction. He nearly relapsed several times, but his guilt and anger with himself for giving in helped to put him back on the right road. He has regained Sandra's confidence, stays away from casinos, card games, and betting parlors, and at last feels able to get on with his life.

OTHER EMOTIONAL PROBLEMS

Serious emotional problems aren't always self-apparent. Many people need a professional diagnosis before they can understand the true cause of disturbance in their lives.

There are a number of emotional and psychological aberrations that can affect people without their realizing they have a problem. Many individuals suffer symptoms that are difficult to identify with a specific condition or that might not be recognized as part of a disorder; examples are excessive dependency on a loved one and extreme reactions to particular ideas. Only recently have doctors begun to see certain behavior patterns as symptoms of emotional problems. Because psychological difficulties can affect an entire family, both in terms of stress and self-denial, therapists are increasingly understanding the need for treatment to involve the whole family.

CODEPENDENCY

Feelings of allegiance as well as personal needs can often make conflicting and difficult demands on an individual. Some people find themselves in a situation that they realize will involve painful confrontations or disruption of comfortable routines in order to do what is best for a partner or loved one. Living with an alcoholic, for example, presents a series of problems for the whole family, and confronting a loved one with disapproval can lead to even further disruption.

Many people find it easier to put up with the consequences of a strained relationship, deciding that what little security there is has greater appeal than confronting and dealing with more serious problems. In fact, there is evidence to suggest that some people feel the only sense of control they have derives from the addict's dependence on them. In this sense the partner is as emotionally dependent on his or her loved one as the addict is dependent on a substance. While the long-term risks—for example, ill health, physical abuse, or the potential destruction of the family home—are far greater, the immediate desire for a relatively stable environment and the sense of being depended on for emotional support somehow seem more important. In such cases a person's insecurity and need for the partner becomes greater than the desire to see the partner well, happy, and independent. The personal, perhaps selfish requirements of one person override the other person's need for real help and some constructive guidance.

Such emotional dependency can itself be destructive because both addict and codependent get caught in a cycle of self-destructive behavior. In extreme cases, it can be possible for a person to make a loved one increasingly dependent on him or her. By pursuing all kinds of exploitative behavior, such as using words or actions that induce a feeling of guilt, a person can make a loved one unable to confront the truth. While this can help to reinforce immediate feelings of security and fulfilled needs, it does so under a false set of values and is essentially destructive to all involved.

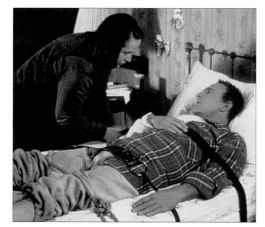

DESPERATE MEASURES
In the tense movie thriller Misery, *a disturbed book fan, Annie Wilkes, attempts to satisfy her emotional need to be in control by holding her favorite author captive. By progressively injuring him both physically and mentally, she makes his very survival utterly dependent on her.*

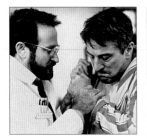

CATATONIC SCHIZOPHRENIA
Some of the bizarre manifestations of catatonic schizophrenia were brought to light in the film Awakenings. *The disorder often leaves a person in a frozen posture and sleeplike condition for long periods of time.*

SCHIZOPHRENIA

Schizophrenia is not a very common disorder, affecting only about 1 percent of the population, but the disease involves a split between the individual's inner and outer realities that can be very debilitating. Symptoms in acute cases include hallucinations, delusions about power or of being pursued by malicious forces, and hearing "voices in the head." Many sufferers respond to situations with inappropriate behavior, perhaps smiling at bad news or failing to respond at all.

Proper medical care is essential; people with acute forms of the disease may harm themselves or others. Hospitalization is often necessary during an acute attack, but with appropriate medications, therapeutic support, and rehabilitation, many patients can lead fairly normal lives, especially if they avoid the stresses that can trigger an attack.

The cause of schizophrenia is unknown, but those who treat it believe that a combination of inherited and environmental factors is involved. It may be a genetic disorder because it tends to run in families.

OBSESSIVE-COMPULSIVE DISORDER

Obsessive-compulsive disorder is characterized by persistent and unwanted thoughts and fears that cause anxiety. The thoughts

DISSOCIATIVE IDENTITY DISORDER

Dissociative identity disorder, or split personality, as it is more commonly known, is a rare condition in which a person possesses two or more distinct personalities. Some of these identities are more dominant than others, alternately taking control of the individual's behavior. Significantly, people with this condition also appear to experience selective amnesia, often failing to retain information that they learn when under the spell of one personality and claiming complete ignorance of their other selves. The cause of the disorder is still unknown, although one theory suggests that people use multiple personalities to distance themselves from painful memories of early life.

that enter the mind of obsessive people are often subjectively absurd, offensive, or irrational, but so compelling that it is difficult to override them. Many sufferers resort to compulsive behavior—repetitive, ritualistic acts such as checking several times that windows are locked or washing their hands excessively—in an attempt to reassure themselves that all is well. These rituals momentarily and superficially reduce their anxiety.

Some patients develop superstitious beliefs that they are convinced will help prevent misfortune. Performing a certain task in a particular way, for example, or following a rigid routine often helps an individual to feel some sense of control. A disruption in this routine is very upsetting and reinforces the ritualistic performance. Most people develop minor obsessions or compulsions at some point in their lives; it is only when the thoughts and actions become so persistent they interfere with normal life that the condition becomes a disorder.

Treatment for obsessive-compulsive disorders range from mild antidepressants and tranquilizers to psychological behavior therapies. Medications relieve some of the symptoms, but only therapy can get at the underlying fear that is causing them. Many patients have been cured by a process similar to that for dealing with phobias (see

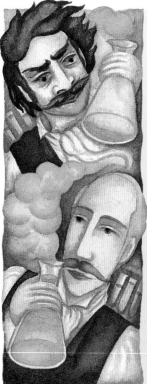

Fables and behavior

DR. JEKYLL AND MR. HYDE

Robert Louis Stevenson's famous tale *The Strange Case of Dr. Jekyll and Mr. Hyde* has entered Western culture as a symbol of split personality. In fact, the story is an effective portrayal of how some individuals tend to repress their true character until it finally emerges with full and potent effect.

Dr. Jekyll, an apparently virtuous man, has spent so much of his life repressing his natural instincts that when he discovers a potion to release his "inner self," the creature Mr. Hyde emerges to take over. Jekyll's inability to control Hyde suggests that we should all acknowledge the good and bad in ourselves to establish a healthy balance and attain self-enlightenment.

A Compulsive Hand Washer

Obsessive-compulsive disorders can take strange and apparently bewildering forms that affect not only the sufferer but also family members and friends. Compulsive washing is a typical example of the condition and is particularly distressing when it becomes so acute that it affects the sufferer's ability to function normally in daily life.

Tom is a 20-year-old student who is obsessed with cleanliness. He is convinced that anything he touches in a public place is dirty and covered with germs. Tom never uses a toilet in a bar or restaurant, and even at home he washes his hands often and for a long time.

Tom feels extremely anxious and uncomfortable if he is forced to stand or sit by other people for extended periods. He wears gloves when reading college library books and never touches door handles with his bare hands. The obsession is beginning to affect his entire life. His friends cannot understand his behavior and feel that he is becoming antisocial. Although Tom knows that he has a problem, he doesn't know what to do about it.

WHAT SHOULD TOM DO?

Tom is suffering from an obsession about contamination that is reflected in his compulsive behavior. There is a danger that, if left untreated, his compulsive habits will seriously interfere with his studies and disrupt his social life.

Tom's obsessive-compulsive disorder is too advanced to be treated by self-help; he needs to get professional psychological support. His doctor can refer him to a psychiatrist, who may work with a cognitive behavior therapist to treat Tom's problem directly. Together they will help Tom to figure out what lies behind his fear, to try to see his fear in a more rational light, and to relearn the behavior patterns that are interfering with his life.

Action Plan

EMOTIONAL HEALTH
Professional guidance can help in finding the underlying cause of this distressing disorder and to overcome abnormal and disruptive behavior patterns.

LIFESTYLE
Be open about problems, particularly with friends and family, in order to enlist their help and support.

PERSONAL HYGIENE
Deal with the practical problems of the disorder by monitoring excessive behavior, perhaps using a diary or making notes.

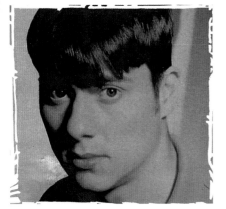

PERSONAL HYGIENE
Personal hygiene is important, but taken too far, it can be disruptive to normal life.

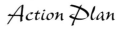

EMOTIONAL HEALTH
Emotional and mental disorders can be very troubling and difficult to cope with.

LIFESTYLE
Maladaptive behavior can affect social life and inhibit personal development and enjoyment.

HOW THINGS TURNED OUT FOR TOM

Tom underwent extensive behavior therapy, discussing his discomforts and feelings of disgust and learning how to change inappropriate conduct. The therapist encouraged Tom to work toward some targets, gradually reducing the number of times he washes his hands and the time spent on each washing. As he better controlled his compulsion, Tom began to feel more comfortable about going out and started to socialize more.

FALSE IMAGES
Dolls with an obviously unrealistic figure like this one have been blamed for setting false ideals of body image in young people's minds.

pages 107–109), in which they are taught that nothing negative happens when a compulsive act is not performed. By learning to postpone a certain behavior for increasing periods of time, a patient should be able to avoid it altogether eventually.

EATING DISORDERS

Obesity can be a serious threat to physical health, but eating disorders like anorexia and bulimia can be equally damaging. Although these conditions are essentially psychological in origin, they can seriously undermine physical health. Anorexia, characterized by dangerously low food intake, and bulimia, which involves binge eating followed by self-induced vomiting, can both lead to nutritional deficiencies and other health problems.

Anorexia and bulimia

Sufferers of anorexia often have a distorted self-image and will constantly try to reduce their body weight, refusing to accept advice that they are already excessively thin. If the condition is not addressed, the body will suffer from malnutrition and stop functioning normally, reducing the heart rate and perhaps disrupting the menstrual cycle.

Sufferers of bulimia have an extreme sense of guilt about their eating and so tend to follow each binge by vomiting or taking laxatives. By immediately removing food from the body after a binge, the individual fails to receive the nutrition that the body needs and so can suffer not only from malnutrition but also other conditions of poor health.

There are several theories about why people develop eating disorders. Researchers agree that cultural factors relating to the ideal body image play some part, but this does not explain why only certain people suffer. Following experiments with rats, some scientists now believe that the hypothalamus, the part of the brain that controls eating and appetite, can partly determine an individual's predisposition to eating disorders. If the gland is dysfunctional and that person is vulnerable to media influences, he or she may develop an eating problem. Therapists now work toward stabilizing a patient's diet while also using cognitive therapy to address the underlying psychological cause.

HELPING A TEENAGER TO LEARN TO LIKE HER BODY

The physical changes of puberty often can lead to a heightened sense of dissatisfaction with one's own body, and media images of super-slim models can make this hard to deal with, especially for young women. Many teenage girls are self-conscious about their bodily changes, and unrealistic ideals accentuate their discomfort. Although some girls are more prone to obsession with such images than others, there is much you can do to help your daughter come to terms with her body and learn to accept the way she looks and feels.

▶ *Encourage your daughter to take up or continue with an exercise or sport that she enjoys and that will keep her healthy. This will help her stay in good physical shape, which can boost confidence and self-esteem and also provide social opportunities.*

▶ *Having a massage can be an excellent way of learning to relax and enjoy your body. You could perhaps suggest that mother and daughter go to a massage session together, and this will provide the perfect opportunity to spend time in relaxing intimacy.*

▶ *Encourage your youngster to take long, therapeutic baths with aromatherapy oils. The relaxing environment will help her to get rid of tension and increasingly accept the changes in her body.*

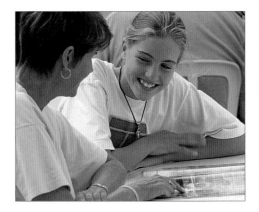

OPEN DISCUSSION
Talking to your teenage daughter about what is happening to her and how she feels about it can help her to accept her changing body.

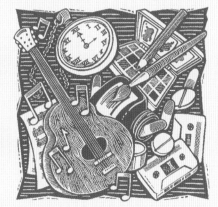

THERAPIES FOR MENTAL HEALTH

*A number of different therapies aim to restore
mental balance and address emotional disorders.
Some involve conventional medical and psychiatric
approaches, whereas others incorporate a whole
range of creative and expressive techniques to help
individuals return to good mental health.*

THE BENEFITS OF THERAPY

Many therapies are available for improving mental and emotional health. While some aim to resolve specific problems, others are geared toward general improvement.

Everybody feels deeply distressed or anxious at times, but the point at which they might need therapy is difficult to determine. While it might be obvious that a person suffering from paranoid schizophrenia needs immediate attention, other mental problems can be harder to identify and resolve. Psychological research suggests that we purposely repress certain anxieties and emotions, and reidentifying these underlying problems can be difficult.

If we have made an unconscious effort to deny our true feelings, how can we expect to acknowledge them readily and confront them as causes of further emotional imbalance? Uncovering hidden problems may require the help of a professional therapist who is skilled in objective analysis and who has the knowledge and insight to determine whether a problem really constitutes a serious disorder.

WHO NEEDS THERAPY?

There is no simple answer to the question of who requires therapy; mental health specialists themselves sometimes disagree over the type and seriousness of conditions that need treatment. A psychotherapist might say that a certain mental condition involves latent anxieties and fears that require professional help, whereas a holistic therapist might see everyday stress as something that needs to be counteracted in order to live life to the fullest. The point at which people feel dis-

---

PSYCHOLOGICAL DISORDERS

Theorists have argued for years about what defines a psychological disorder. While some people associate only extreme problems like schizophrenia with the term, others might include phobias or inhibitions that greatly restrict a person from living a full life.

Professionals tend to define disorders according to the type of abnormality in behavior and feeling. Defining what actually *is* normal can present some difficulty, but a person suffering from any of the following problems probably needs some kind of help.

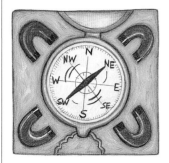

FEELING LOST *Anyone who suffers constant anxiety, depression, fear, or confusion is probably feeling lost.*

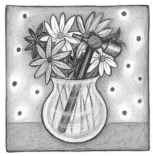

ATYPICALITY *Behavior that is bizarrely different from that of other people is considered atypical.*

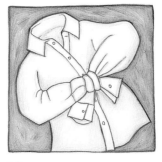

MALADAPTIVENESS *Any behavior that interferes with a person's normal functioning is maladaptive.*

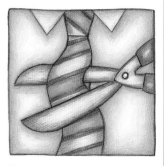

DISRUPTIVENESS *Behavior that interferes with normal social intercourse and routines is disruptive.*

Origins

Treatment for people with severe mental disorders was extremely harsh until the 19th century. Patients were often shackled in dark, unsanitary cells or restrained with various contraptions. One example of such an apparatus was the "circulatory swing," a hoist in which the patient was suspended from the ceiling and spun around (see illustration, right).

In 1793 Parisian Philipe Pinel argued that the treatment for mental disorders should be revised. Believing that patients needed kindness rather than harsh treatment, he campaigned to move them to more humane environments and opened a large hospital in Paris that year. His new regimen produced impressive results, with many patients apparently recovering. Although it is likely that many of Pinel's hospitalized patients had only minor disturbances rather than serious mental illnesses, his colleagues were still sufficiently impressed to agree to revise their own practices. Compassionate therapy at last began to replace repression.

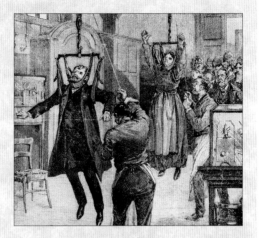

CIRCULATORY SWING
This crude device was used to spin patients. It was thought that the ensuing dizziness and disorientation helped to restore mental order.

tress enough that they need assistance is largely up to them to decide, unless they become so troubled that close family members have to make the decision.

Denying your emotions or pretending that you do not need help when you do can be dangerous. If you ever feel that stress is affecting your health or that your life has lost direction, you should talk your anxieties through with a close friend or family member. If this does not seem to help, then talk to a doctor, counselor, or social worker who is willing to listen to problems and can recommend therapies and support groups that may help. Remember that seeking help is a sign of personal strength and control rather than one of weakness.

CHOOSING YOUR THERAPY

Your doctor or a counselor may recommend a particular therapy, or you may decide to consult a specialist without any referral. Because there is a vast array of therapies to choose from, it is important to know exactly what you want to achieve. Assessing whether you have a serious emotional problem or simply would like to get progressively more in touch with your feelings is a sensible way to begin the selection process. Personal recommendations about a therapist can be useful, but remember that what works for one person will not necessarily work for another individual.

Ultimately, you can achieve real mental balance only if you are committed to your personal development. Resistance or skeptical dismissal of a particular therapy indicates that you may not have the necessary desire or will to make it work.

THE FIRST CONSULTATION

Before deciding whether to pursue a particular therapy, it is a good idea to meet with the practitioner and have him or her explain in everyday language what the sessions will be like, how often you will need to meet, and what kind of issues you are likely to be exploring. Talking through what your anxieties are, what you want therapy to achieve, and any apprehensions you have about counseling can help you determine whether you have found the right therapist.

As you discuss the long-term plan, ask yourself the following questions:

▶ *Do I feel a rapport between us?*

▶ *Would I feel comfortable disclosing personal information to this person?*

▶ *Do I feel that this therapist would be able to understand the situation I am in?*

▶ *Am I confident that this person would never take advantage of my emotional vulnerability?*

▶ *Do I feel that this person has the ability to help me?*

PSYCHOTHERAPY

The most familiar treatment for mental and emotional health involves some kind of psychotherapy in which a therapist helps an individual to identify and deal with anxieties.

The term *psychotherapy* covers a broad range of treatments for many different problems. Essentially, however, it refers to the use of psychological techniques, such as a discussion of feelings, to treat emotional, behavioral, and interpersonal problems. It offers the opportunity for anyone who feels depressed to talk to a specialist in a safe and secure environment. Away from the normal routine of relationships and social networks, individuals can discuss anything from bereavement to rejection to inhibition. Radical changes in a person's life can bring on great stress and the inability to cope with it, so learning to examine and express deep-seated feelings can go a long way toward relieving anxiety.

HOW PSYCHOTHERAPY CAN HELP

The specific ways in which psychotherapy is able to help a person will vary, but there are several general principles. Initially, meetings with a therapist will be used to help the patient understand the actual problem. While the patient might suggest that there is one particular source of anxiety, for example, the therapist will encourage further exploration so that a more complete picture emerges. This might mean discussing issues

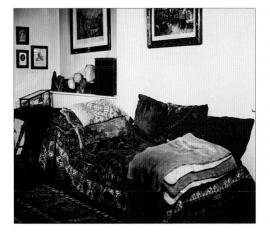

FREUD'S COUCH
When treating patients, Freud famously asked them to lie back on a couch. The intention was to help them relax and feel able to discuss anxieties openly.

> **CAUTION**
> *Psychological therapy and counseling provide mechanisms for dealing with life's challenges; they are not an alternative to living life itself. It is important not to replace the search for meaningful relationships with a series of weekly one-hour therapy sessions.*

and thoughts that appear to have no direct connection with the problem at hand. A therapist needs to get to know his or her patient as fully as possible in order to decide whether the mind is suppressing some emotional impulse or disturbance that the patient is unaware of.

Psychotherapeutic sessions provide a safe space in which the client can talk openly and at length. Feeling secure in the knowledge that the therapist will not judge what they are saying, people are often at their most open and expressive in these sessions, releasing pent-up emotions and relieving stress. The detached but informed and sympathetic professional can encourage a relationship of trust, which enables the therapist and patient to work together. While psychotherapists resist giving direct advice, they usually encourage their clients to explore new ways of looking at their difficulties and finding solutions for themselves.

The nonreciprocal nature of the relationship is important. Although the client can expect support, insight, and sympathetic listening from the therapist, he or she does not need to reciprocate this compassion. While such completely honest discussion and self-reflection might put strain on a friendship, the client can enjoy the same supportive framework without the emotional risk. If it is effective, counseling and support provide the security of friendship without potentially jeopardizing or putting excessive burden on normal, interactive relationships.

PSYCHOANALYTIC THERAPY

Psychoanalysis originated in Vienna in the late 19th century with Sigmund Freud. His ideas have been enormously influential in all areas of psychotherapy and even in general Western thought. Freud revised his ideas throughout his lifetime, and many of those who followed his teachings also developed some of the concepts further, a few of them even branching out into opposing factions in the process. Alfred Adler, Wilhelm Reich, and Carl Jung, for example, began their careers as Freudian disciples before going on to develop and contest many psychoanalytic theories. Nevertheless, the contribution that Freud made toward modern psychotherapy is incalculable.

Classical psychoanalysis is founded on the idea that, in terms of the working mind, conscious awareness is only the tip of the

FREUD'S INTERPRETATION OF DREAMS

Freud believed that desires and impulses find an outlet in dreams through the use of particular imagery. Any repressed anxieties about sex, for example, are said to be symbolized in common, everyday objects. Sharp objects, such as swords, represent the phallus, while containers and enclosed spaces symbolize the womb. Going up or descending stairs is said to reflect the sexual act.

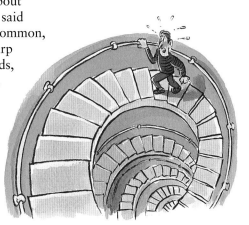

SEXUAL SYMBOLS
Freud claimed that our inner tensions, such as anxiety about sex, are displaced onto everyday images and activities like climbing stairs.

WHO'S WHO?

The distinctions between different mental health professionals can be confusing. The following brief definitions are a basic guide to these differences.

▶ *Psychiatrists are physicians (M.D.s) who specialize in mental disorders. As doctors they have the authority to prescribe medication, and many specialize in talking-based psychotherapy.*

▶ *Psychologists have training and usually advanced degrees in psychotherapy but cannot prescribe medications.*

▶ *Clinical psychologists have training in psychotherapies but most often work in research and personality assessment.*

▶ *Psychiatric nurses have basic nursing training plus postgraduate studies with a special focus on mental health. These professionals usually work in hospitals or psychiatric units.*

▶ *Psychoanalysts, who may or may not have medical degrees, generally follow conventional Freudian theories on therapy and have themselves been psychoanalyzed. They tend to be involved in one-on-one consultations rather than in a team.*

iceberg. Freud argued that underlying the world of consciousness is a deeper, subconscious level to which we have no immediate access. While the conscious mind works on normal, logical principles, the subconscious is driven by emotional links, using symbols and associations to formulate and express concepts. So while we are thinking on the conscious level, the underlying motivation for these thoughts can be considerably more complex and profound.

According to Freud, only through accessing the subconscious can a therapist discover the true cause of a person's emotional disorder or anxiety. Freud's form of psychotherapy was designed to help identify and release these repressed conflicts in a different and healthier form. Because the subconscious is essentially unexpressed, Freud believed that the mind uses certain behaviors and images to articulate inner thought.

With the use of such techniques as hypnosis or free word association, a patient would be encouraged to relax and allow the mind to wander naturally, thus allowing these images and symbols to surface. Unintentional behavior, such as slips of the tongue, or "Freudian slips," is said to reveal what a person is really thinking below the level of current conversation.

One of Freud's most famous techniques was interpretation of dreams. He believed that the subconscious is at its most active

continued on page 126

Your Dreams

There are many techniques for and books on dream analysis. However, you do not need extensive training to analyze your own dreams; learning to record them and interpret recurring images may help you resolve some ongoing problems.

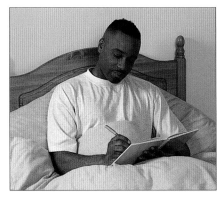

DREAM RECALL
As you wake up, lie quietly for a while and think of all of the images and sensations that you experienced in your dream. Then write them down as fully as possible.

Many people claim they do not remember dreaming while they were asleep. However, researchers believe that we may have as many as five or six dreams each night. With practice, it is possible to learn how to remember and document them so that you can later analyze their images and symbolic meaning. One key step is to develop the confidence that you *will* be able to recall images and then focus your attention. As you wake up, lie still for a while and concentrate on whatever ideas or emotions have emerged from your sleep. Then write down everything you can remember, from main themes to minor details, and also note any emotions or associations that you feel. After several weeks of daily recording and practice, you should start to see some dream patterns emerging, and your skills of recall should improve.

COMMON DREAM INTERPRETATIONS

In order to interpret dreams effectively, you need to understand how your subconscious processes ideas. According to Freud's theories (see page 123) and ideas about dreams, objects and images often operate as symbols in them and rarely have literal meaning. The image of an empty purse, for example, may reflect loss of security and love rather than a more predictable interpretation of worries over finance. Similarly, holding a dinner party or cooking for other people in a dream may suggest that the dreamer wishes to influence others or mold some truth into a more palatable form. Understanding how your mind shapes its subconscious into visual images will help you to identify and interpret certain characteristics of it.

TIPS FOR REMEMBERING DREAMS

▶ *Avoid alcohol or caffeine before going to sleep because these reduce REM (rapid eye movement)—the period of sleep during which most dreaming occurs.*

▶ *Keep a paper and pencil or, better still, a tape recorder beside your bed for recording dreams.*

▶ *Try to avoid using an alarm clock. People usually wake up naturally just after dreaming.*

▶ *Keep your eyes closed as you think about a dream to prevent external stimuli from interfering.*

▶ *Date each dream and review your records once a month to identify recurring patterns.*

CONDENSATION
The term condensation *refers to an image or idea that is made up of several others. A number of different people may be represented in one single dream character, for example, or several objects may become condensed into one. Theorists believe that this is the mind's way of diluting the threatening nature of any one of the people or objects represented. For example, a dream character might have the clothes of your brother, the face of your boss, and the voice of your ex-lover—a condensation of people who may have dominated you at some point in your life.*

DISPLACEMENT

Displacement refers to a distinct shift of focus between latent, unacknowledged anxieties and those that are brought to the surface. Extreme fears or conflicts might manifest themselves in a dream as less threatening objects or events. Subconscious anger toward a person, for example, might cause the dreamer to imagine damaging an object belonging to this figure rather than acting violently toward the person.

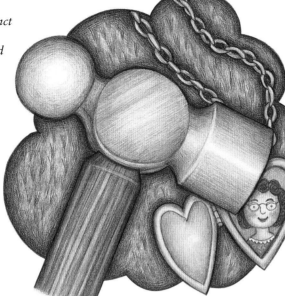

RECURRING FEATURES

Many of the common aspects in dreams have particular psychological interpretations.

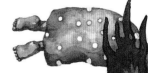

FLYING

In addition to sexual desire, flying may also suggest a sense of freedom and insight. This contrasts with the more disturbing sensation of falling, which implies that a person is anxious about achievement. Kite flying suggests a controlled freedom.

PERSONIFICATION

Personification occurs when an abstract or complex anxiety is represented as a particular individual. Worry about a test, for example, might be personified in a dream by the presence of a teacher. Anxiety about growing old might be personified by a grandfather, and fear of sexual inadequacy might be represented by the appearance of a stereotypically sexy film star.

NUDITY

While anxiety about nudity might reflect a fear of being seen as one really is, accepting the nakedness of others indicates an ability to see through people's defenses. Disgust at nudity suggests displeasure in discovering another person's real self.

SOME COMMON DREAM THEMES

Although symbolism in dreams is largely personal and idiosyncratic, there are certain events and images that occur in many people's dreams and that therapists associate with particular latent thoughts. Flying can be an expression of sexual desire or, more generally, a desire for freedom. Being nude in public is often interpreted as a fear of being seen as one really is. Falling suggests that an individual may have climbed too high in personal or professional life and anticipates a metaphorical tumble. Being chased suggests that there are aspects of the unseen self that are clamoring for release into the consciousness. The dreamer's fear often dissolves if he or she is able to turn around in the dream, thus confronting the self and overcoming self-repression.

Males tend to dream about men rather than women, which possibly underlines the role of competitiveness in male anxiety. Women, however, tend to dream about the sexes equally, revealing the significance of relationships for them.

RUNNING AWAY

Trying to run away from an unseen presence indicates that a person is trying to avoid confronting or admitting some personal anxieties or inhibitions. Turning to face the pursuer can often dissipate the fear.

125

THE THREE DIVISIONS OF SELF

According to Freudian psychoanalysis three mental structures comprise the personality. The id, which is entirely subconscious, embodies our innate instincts of sex and aggression. Because these impulses are deemed socially unacceptable, however, we repress the id with the ego—the conscious self that controls and directs our contact with reality. The superego starts developing at about the age of five and is the moral force that we learn to live by. Freud believed good mental health involves a happy balance among all three aspects.

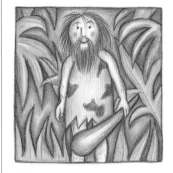

THE ID
The embodiment of our natural impulses, the id involves our innate instincts.

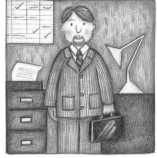

THE EGO
We use the conscious ego to assert respectability and repress the instincts of the id.

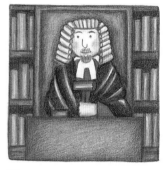

THE SUPEREGO
Our moral force, the superego sets the standards by which we live.

when the conscious mind is asleep, allowing real desires and impulses to roam in the mind and articulate themselves in the form of dream images. Freud spent a lot of time trying to interpret dreams, believing that these symbols were the key to understanding an individual's subconscious. Because the images are created by the subconscious, they are often more complex and profound than first appears. For example, an individual might think that a dream about an old man reflects an encounter earlier that day, while Freud might see such a dream figure as symbolic of the patient's father. In essence, he believed that everybody displaces and transfers subconscious thoughts and needs into other, more manageable images.

The question of how such inner turmoil is allowed to build up and infiltrate the conscious is an interesting one. Freud placed great emphasis on the importance of childhood experiences and believed that innate sexual passion and unarticulated emotion in these formative years cause tension that gets locked up in the cellar of the mind. Such conflicts and their associated anxieties do not stay passively repressed, however. Their psychological "energy" is so strong that they must constantly seek ways out of the subconscious and into responsive awareness. Taking the form of inhibition, anxiety, or other emotional problems, the troubled subconscious struggles against the repressive conscious, causing internal conflict and disturbed behavior. Freud's work, therefore,

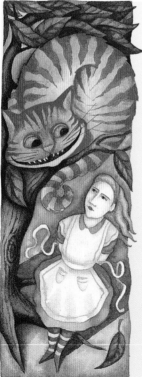

Fables and myths

ALICE IN WONDERLAND

Lewis Carroll's classic children's story *Alice's Adventures in Wonderland* depicts the journey of a little girl through a number of strange and enlightening encounters. Famous for its apparently nonsensical characters, the story actually encourages us to reassess many of our literal assumptions. The grinning Cheshire Cat, for example, or Alice's hosts at the tea party all present absurd deviations from conventional expectations of behavior and interaction. Alice's trip is an allegorical journey in which social convention is constantly questioned. After confronting the many absurdities of existence, she becomes better reconciled with her thoughts and more socially aware.

involved accepting that internal turmoil and repression are part of common existence but that excessive conflict can be emotionally destructive. Although he was often ridiculed for his emphasis on sex, and though some of his theories are difficult to prove, Freud is still credited today with developing much of our understanding of the human psyche.

HUMANISTIC THERAPY

Whereas Freud believed that psychological disorders stem from unresolved inner conflicts, humanistic theorists believe that they arise through environmental interference to personal growth and fulfillment. For them the heart of therapy lies in encouraging patients to find personal meaning in life and to live in ways that are consistent with their individual traits and personalities. A number of different therapies are based on humanistic beliefs, all of which emphasize the positive impulses of human nature.

Rogerian therapy

Carl Rogers devised a client-centered therapy in the 1970s and 1980s. It works on the principle that only the client really knows what his or her problem is and what the realistic options are for responding to it. Rather than directing a counseling session, practitioners seek to provide a positive therapeutic climate and display a genuine interest in a person's problems. By empathizing with the patient, the therapist attempts to see and feel the world from a similar perspective, provide unconditional regard, and avoid passing judgment.

Rogerian therapists perceive the main cause of psychological stress to be a mismatch between self-concept and reality. In general, they believe that individuals suffer emotional conflict when they overvalue the approval of others and lack self-esteem. It is thus important to help patients realize their own personal growth by encouraging self-acceptance and personal values.

Gestalt therapy

Gestalt therapy had a huge impact on the development of mental treatment in the 1960s and 1970s. Emphasizing a freedom to experience and express emotions, the principles of the therapy fitted in well with the cultural movements of its heyday. The term *gestalt* comes from the German *gestalten* and means "whole things," emphasizing

GESTALT THERAPY Patients are encouraged to role-play situations, perhaps using furniture as a stand-in for a key person, thus acting out their impulses and emotions.

the importance of awareness in perception and the wholeness of experience. Fritz Perls, the originator of this psychotherapy, claimed that individuals experience emotional difficulties because they refuse to acknowledge, or they effectively disown, parts of their own being. To rectify this situation, therapists may directly challenge a client's behavior or ask him or her to portray unresolved conflicts. This role play with objects can range from talking to an empty chair that personifies an authoritarian figure to using lightweight bats to hit objects and safely express anger. Other innovative techniques include marathon sessions in which clients work nonstop at expressing their emotions for two to three days. The theory is that as fatigue and emotional exhaustion take effect, some psychological defense mechanisms become weakened and significant progress can be made.

COGNITIVE THERAPY

Cognitive therapy is a process of probing for insight that focuses on changing negative thinking habits. It assumes that psychological distress is caused by distorted modes of thought, such as biased inferences, and

CARL ROGERS One of the founders of humanistic therapy, Rogers identified a number of different thinking patterns.

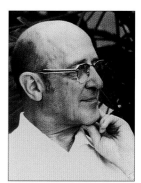

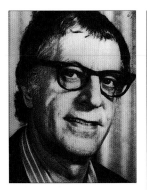

ALBERT ELLIS
The founder of rational emotive therapy (RET), Albert Ellis took cognitive therapy one step further and promoted the value of positive and objective thinking.

basic errors of logic and deduction. In other words, what we think strongly affects how we feel and what we do. A number of therapists have refined these principles to construct their own cognitive therapies.

Beck's cognitive therapy

A leader in the development of cognitive therapy (also called cognitive behavior therapy), Aaron Beck identified several negative thinking habits that he suggested lead to a pessimistic outlook and, potentially, full-blown depression. One common habit, self-referencing, is built on the assumption that you are the focus of everyone else's negative feelings and actions. Overgeneralizing is assuming that the negative consequences of one instance apply to all other situations. Catastrophizing is simply taking for granted that the worst will always happen. Selective abstraction results from focusing only on negative evidence that affirms your fears.

Although Beck's therapy does not disprove the irrationality of these tendencies, patients are invited to explore their thinking habits. Individuals look at how they make assumptions about themselves and discuss why they pursue self-defeating thoughts. Cognitive therapists help their patients to reappraise any negative thought processes through discussion and by testing out new ideas in performing homework assignments. Unlike psychoanalytic psychotherapy, the main emphasis is on the present, although relevant past experiences will be discussed. (See pages 104, 108, 109, and117 for information on uses of cognitive therapy.)

Rational emotive therapy

Rational emotive therapy, or RET, as it is often called, focuses on the assumptions that provide the basis for a client's anxiety and depression. While it is similar to Beck's cognitive theories, this therapy aims to demonstrate and persuade a patient how irrational and badly distorted some of his or her perceptions are. By questioning the motivation behind a self-deprecating comment, the therapist helps a person to confront the unhelpful ways of thinking that undermine the search for happiness. Albert Ellis, who devised RET, believed that cognitive assumptions actually intervene between external events and emotional reactions. By drawing a direct link between irrational assumptions and emotional responses, therapists encourage their patients to develop habits of positive thinking and objective rationality.

POSITIVE THINKING

Thinking positively and leaving troubles behind can be difficult to do. Although serious problems should always be treated by a professional therapist, there are visualizations you can do by yourself to improve your state of mind. The following visualization can encourage a positive perspective, helping you focus on the present rather than the past. This transformation will help provide confidence to face the future.

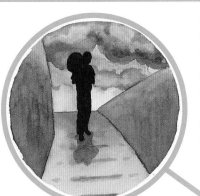

As you move into the tunnel, the dark and eerie silence feels a little oppressive, but you continue your journey. As you walk along, old doubts and regrets come to the surface of your mind, reminding you of failures, mistakes, and missed opportunities. As they surface, however, your bag begins to feel a little lighter, and these regrets are gradually set free from your mind.

Imagine yourself walking along a gray, flat path. High banks on either side and a cloudy sky above make you feel heavy and make your footsteps slow. You are carrying a bag, and its weight causes your back to bend as you approach a damp and dark tunnel.

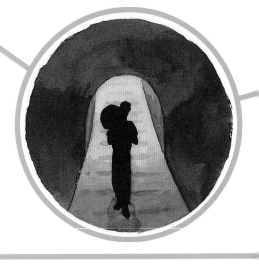

HYPNOTHERAPY

Although hypnotherapy went through a phase of negative publicity when it was used as entertainment, its professional value as a treatment remains important. Many people have successfully overcome addictions, bad habits, or physical and emotional problems with the help of hypnosis.

Hypnotherapy works by calming the conscious mind so that the patient can attain a trancelike state and focus completely on the therapist's suggestions. In this deep state of relaxation, the therapist can then reinforce a person's positive attitudes, encourage self-belief, or cause muscles that are involuntarily tense to relax.

Hypnotherapy has shown amazing results in treating physiological conditions, such as high blood pressure and asthma, as well as problems like anxiety. Recent work by a gastroenterologist in Manchester, England, demonstrated an extraordinary 80 percent success rate for hypnotherapy in the treatment of irritable bowel syndrome. It is thought that through complete relaxation and the patient's desire to be cured, the mind is more open to those suggestions that it already seeks. In other words, hypnosis sets up the framework for self-cure, encouraging confidence in the self as a healer. During a procedure patients are always aware of what is going on and are in control of their activities and behavior; they are able to wake up at any time.

GROUP AND FAMILY THERAPY

In group therapy one or more therapists work with several people at the same time. By sharing experiences, individuals can sympathetically challenge each others' views and perceptions, developing a sense of team solidarity. Conditions from alcoholism to bereavement to abuse can all be treated with group therapy, which may be led by either a professional or a fellow sufferer.

Family therapy is designed to assist the entire family unit when one member has been identified as having a psychological problem. It is based on the idea that family systems, rather than individual family members, can be at fault and that everybody needs to address the underlying cause. For example, sending out conflicting messages, such as saying that you forgive someone but then avoiding that person, can cause immense pressure within the family. Therapists help families to assess and improve their methods of communication.

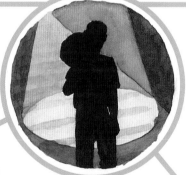

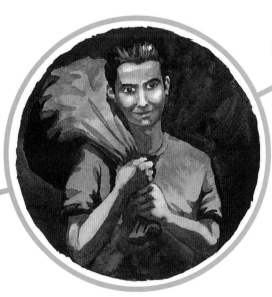

Walking suddenly into a pool of light, you remember a happy incident, a time when you laughed and felt good about yourself.

Moving back into the darkness, you feel the bag lightening even further as more regrets come to mind. Your back becomes a little straighter as the surfacing doubts increasingly relieve the load. Another pool of light and another recollection of pleasure help you to feel better before going back into the darkness.

Approaching the end of the tunnel, you feel the warmth and light of the midday sun. Your steps are much lighter as you walk toward this brightness; your bag is empty and your mind feels fresh. Stepping out into the sun, you feel enthusiastic about all of the adventures ahead of you and free of the inhibiting emotions and regrets that have been holding you down.

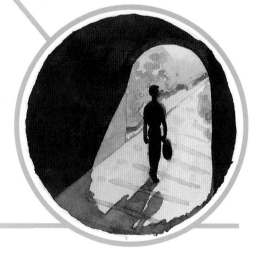

An Insecure Woman

Everyone is sensitive to the comments and observations of people around them, but some individuals become excessively dependent on the approval of others. Needing affirmation in everything you do can limit your personal growth and lead to a profound lack of confidence, inhibiting your ability to succeed alone and placing great strain on your relationships.

Anita is 30 and has been dating her boyfriend, Mike, for about two years. Anita would like Mike to move in with her because she feels lonely in her apartment and would like more commitment in their relationship. Mike is reluctant to make such a move, however, because he feels that Anita already depends on him too much. She always seeks his approval on any purchases she makes and constantly offers to run errands for him or help with his work. At her own workplace, Anita insists on taking on extra responsibilities. Every year she organizes the Christmas party alone and takes sole charge of the decorations. It seems she always has to be doing something that demands the attention and approval of others.

WHAT SHOULD ANITA DO?

Anita needs to understand why she must always be busy and seeking people's approval. It seems that she constantly needs reassurance from others because she lacks confidence in her own abilities. Anita could consider seeing a rational emotive therapist (RET), who will encourage her to assess why she needs to organize most of her life around other people. By articulating her ideas about life, Anita can start to question them and consider whether they are always appropriate. Many deep-seated behavior patterns stem from habits adopted in childhood. In order to be happier, Anita needs to start believing in her own worth and establishing her own beliefs and personal goals.

Action Plan

PARTNER
Discuss any problems in the relationship with Mike and assess whether commitments and decisions are being made for the right reasons.

LIFESTYLE
Learn to do things through personal motivation. Make decisions alone as often as possible to develop confidence in abilities and increase independence.

WORK
While it is worthwhile to work hard, don't let a desire to impress others become an obsession.

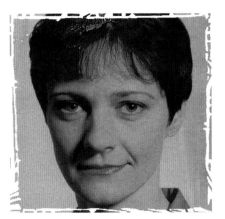

PARTNER
A deep need for constant approval from a partner makes relationships difficult.

LIFESTYLE
Although everybody needs attention and approval, being frightened to make any decisions or assertions alone can be inhibiting.

WORK
Constant striving to make a good impression at work can start to overtake personal life.

HOW THINGS TURNED OUT FOR ANITA

After a series of sessions with an experienced RET therapist, Anita realized that her desire to please others had become too important a part of her life. She and Mike agreed to put off their decision about moving in together for another few months, and Anita made a concerted effort to start developing an independent, social network. She still plans to organize the Christmas party, but has asked for help from other staff members.

BIOMEDICAL THERAPIES

While psychological and humanistic therapies are improving all the time, the role of medication in treating emotional imbalance remains significant as well.

Given the connection between physical and mental health, it is not surprising that some therapies involve biomedical approaches. Many specialists believe that mental disorders, including depression, anxiety, and psychoses like schizophrenia, have some kind of biological origin, and they use drugs or other medical treatment to intervene in the body's natural processes. There is a great deal of controversy over the safety and effectiveness of such treatments and a belief that some are being overprescribed. Still, new drugs are constantly being discovered that specifically target psychological disorders with fewer side effects, and research is increasingly directed at finding the causes rather than just relieving the symptoms of such disorders.

ANTIPSYCHOTIC MEDICATIONS

Antipsychotic drugs can be used for a whole range of psychotic symptoms, including hallucinations and extreme hostility. They work by blocking transmission in the nerve pathways of dopamine, the neurotransmitter in the brain that in excessive amounts has been linked to many psychological problems. The more powerful a drug is in blocking this transmission, the more effective it is in relieving symptoms. Older antipsychotic drugs, like chlorpromazine, caused adverse effects—for example, drowsiness, blurred vision, and Parkinsonian symptoms. Injection of the medication to enable a slower release is now more popular because it is a safer way of applying treatment.

ANTIANXIETY MEDICATIONS

Antianxiety drugs are generally used to aid sleep and relieve stress. The major classes of drugs used to treat this disorder are beta-blockers, which ease physical symptoms, and benzodiazepines, which increase levels of the neurotransmitter gamma-amino-butyric acid (GABA), a brain chemical that normally inhibits brain activity in the part of the brain that controls emotion. Taken in small doses for a limited time, the drugs can be very effective, but prolonged use can affect coordination or lead to addiction. For this reason researchers are now looking for drugs that will lessen anxiety by reducing the impact of the hormone noradrenaline. Because this chemical encourages reactions in the nervous system, scientists believe that inhibiting its activity may lead to a reduction in anxious sensations. While this may prove safer for long-term treatment, no drug will address the real cause of anxiety, which needs to be resolved by the individual with help from a psychotherapist. (See page 104 for information on medications used for treating depression.)

ELECTROCONVULSIVE THERAPY

Electroconvulsive therapy (ECT) is a controversial treatment that is not used as often today as in the past. It involves the use of a general anesthetic to prevent the patient from feeling any pain or remembering the treatment and then a burst of electronic current sent through the brain to induce a brief seizure. Specialists are not sure how the treatment works, but these shocks are effective in treating severe depression and are often favored for patients who have suicidal tendencies. Side effects, such as temporary memory loss for events of the past 6 to 12 months, have caused concern, and controversy over the safety of the treatment has led to ECT being banned in some countries.

Primitive surgery
The earliest theories on mental ill health were concerned with supernatural causes and biological treatment. From the Stone Age until the Renaissance, people generally believed that psychological disorders were caused by evil spirits and possession by demons or witches. Stone Age skulls have been found that contain neatly drilled holes, and these suggest that the surgical procedure of trephining was used to release the evil spirits.

TREPHINED SKULL
The holes in this prehistoric skull may be evidence of early surgery to treat mental disorder.

131

OTHER THERAPIES

*Several mental health therapies that embrace ideas
from various cultures fall outside traditional medical
approaches, but they can still be very beneficial.*

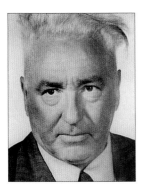

**WILHELM REICH
(1897–1957)**
*Reich was an Austrian
psychoanalyst who
eventually rejected
Freudian principles
for his own theories
on life energy.*

The principle of attaining good emotional balance remains at the center of modern psychological thought. But while mainstream practitioners in mental health primarily talk with patients, treat them with medications, or use a combination of both approaches, there are many alternative therapists who have devised other techniques to help people cope with mental distress. Some of them place much of their emphasis on improving mental well-being through physical expression or release of tensions. Such therapists work toward finding a harmony between mind and body.

REICHIAN THERAPY

Wilhelm Reich broke away from traditional psychoanalysis to develop a therapy that focuses on the relationship of body tension to psychological rigidity. Reichian therapy is based on the idea that we block life energy, or *orgone,* by denying life-affirming emotions, such as joy, anger, sadness, and love, to protect ourselves in response to hurtful and traumatic experiences. He called this process *armoring,* and it is expressed in rigid attitudes, feelings of shame, anxiety, and guilt, and muscular tension.

The goal of orgone therapy is to undo emotional distress by removing armoring. Reich developed exercises that enhance the flow of energy and help restore balance. Breathing, body, voice, and movement exercises, together with supportive touching from the therapist, are used to help the body pull down defensive barriers and release the flow of life energy. Over the course of therapy, a patient replaces chronic pain with more experiences of pleasure and aliveness and develops greater self-esteem.

BODY ALIGNMENT

Rolfers believe that physical and emotional traumas are stored in the body, causing muscles to suffer strain and lose their flexibility. The therapy aims to release stress by realigning the body into its correct posture and to improve functioning. To tell if your body needs help, stand in front of a mirror and imagine a line dropping from the center of your head to the floor. The left and right sides of your body should be balanced. To an observer at your side, your head should ride above the spine, with only shallow curves in the back.

A tilted head
disrupts alignment
in the shoulders.

MISALIGNED
*A curved
spine and
tilted head
suggest poor
posture in
which the
body fails to
function
efficiently and
thus wastes
energy forces.*

An upright neck
prevents strain on
the spine.

ALIGNED
*Upright and
balanced, the
head and
body convey
a positive
posture and
help a person
to reach a
physical and
emotional
optimum.*

ROLFING

One of the therapies that relates stress to dysfunction in the body's structure is Rolfing. Devised by American biochemist Dr. Ida Rolf, the therapy is based on the view that the body is an architectural unit made up of segments, or blocks. When one of these blocks—whether it is the head, shoulders, chest, pelvis, or legs—becomes misaligned, the body is forced to move in a distorted manner, reflecting emotional and physical "dis-ease."

Rolfers believe that memory is stored in both the mind and body, with anxiety and inner turmoil expressing themselves in physical stance. As a therapist vigorously massages the body back into alignment, the individual is able to release emotional conflict and thus become more self-aware.

PRIMAL THERAPY

With roots in psychoanalysis, primal therapy is concerned with appreciating the damaging subtleties of childhood trauma and helping patients to develop new ways of expressing their inner psychic pain. Patients are encouraged to act out and relive primal scenes, or early childhood experiences, until the pool of their various anguishes and pain has been emptied.

In his famous book, *The Primal Scream*, Arthur Janov explains how ultimate relief may come through basic, vocal expression, releasing screams that push out years of emotional suppression and denial. It is common for therapy to be focused on the experience of birth, during which patients are encouraged to adopt the positions and utterances of early stages of physical and emotional development.

Janov claims that working progressively through the emotions of anger, hurt, and love is a reversal of the natural sequence of experiences in life. That is to say, life's progressive path involves being given love, experiencing the hurt of losing it, and then developing anger to ease the pain. Primal therapy works back through these stages, redressing emotional imbalance through hypnosis, breathing techniques, and simulation of the birth experience.

THE ROSEN METHOD

Much like Taoist thoughts on the Three Treasures (see page 145), the Rosen method says that we are born emotionally open and

LOOYENWORK

LooyenWork, developed by Ted Looyen in 1985, is a deep tissue therapy that recognizes a relationship between emotion and posture. Therapists believe that pain or fear expresses itself in the tautness of muscles, and they focus on "reading" the body and trying to "reeducate" it. Using essential oils, the therapist relaxes the muscles with special massage techniques, thereby increasing the flow of energy.

THE EXPRESSIVE BODY Practitioners of LooyenWork believe that tension in different parts of the body reflects specific emotions.

Not being able to express yourself honestly and openly may be reflected in a clenched jaw.

People who are stubborn often suffer from frequent neck pain.

Insecurity may be indicated by tension in the lower back and hips.

An inability to trust other people may be indicated by tight hamstrings.

Anger may be stored in tight and tense calves.

complete. As life progresses, however, we encounter situations in which we are expected to suppress emotion and behave with quiet obedience. Marion Rosen believed that such suppression leads to loss of spontaneity as the muscles become frozen in unnatural holding positions.

Rosen therapists encourage muscular relaxation to help people effectively move out of a contracted body, develop a broader view of life, release emotions, and attain insight. They believe that every individual has muscle aches and tensions that are a kind of chronicle of emotional trauma. By touching different points on the body, the therapist reminds individual muscles that they are holding back and can release some of the tension to which they have become accustomed. As long-imposed muscular tension is relieved, patients often experience emotional liberation. Although the therapy is not suitable for severe emotional disorders or chronic pain, it is often a useful adjunct to other psychotherapies.

continued on page 136

Quindo

Devised to beat stress and boost vitality, Quindo has been heralded as a therapy for the 21st century. Its aim is to give people confidence and a sense of well-being, helping them to gain more control over their own lives.

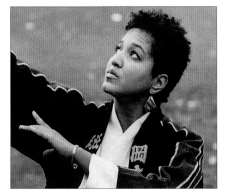

KHALEGHL QUINN
Following martial arts training in Tokyo, psychologist Khaleghl Quinn went on to develop Quindo, which helps people to build confidence and self-esteem.

Quindo is an accessible program of gentle exercises designed to help people achieve their personal best. It was devised by Khaleghl Quinn, a clinical psychologist and martial arts expert, and is based on five simple principles: awareness, strength, confidence, safety, and resilience. Developing the combination of fitness and safety techniques plus relaxation skills enables young and old alike to increase vitality and willpower. By stimulating chi—the body's vital energy—students learn to improve the mind/body connection, gaining confidence in their identities and learning how to assess and constructively counteract stressful situations.

In addition to encouraging skills of self-assertion, Quindo focuses on intuition and self-awareness. Gentle de-stressing techniques and breathing exercises help to balance the nervous system and promote deep relaxation. While practicing, some people choose to wear special wide-legged pants, like those in the following photographs, but any loose, comfortable clothing is appropriate.

THE PUMP

The pump, one of the foundation exercises of Quindo, provides a gentle warm-up, enhancing energy levels and breathing. It is most beneficial if you start slowly, repeating the exercise 10 times, and then build up speed and repetitions using swift, graceful movements. Eventually you should be doing the movements up to 50 times.

1 *Stand with your feet a little more than shoulder width apart, your knees slightly bent, and feet pointing outward. Keep the base of your pelvis beneath the shoulders. Raise your arms to shoulder height, feeling the energy being pulled up through your legs and spine to your head. Hold the position for about 3 seconds.*

2 *Swing the arms downward, allowing the energy to rush through the body. This movement will shift stagnant energy, sending it down into the earth.*

3 *Using the sensitivity of your underarms to guide you, swing your arms back as far as possible without straining. Then swing them forward again to set up a pumping motion. Repeat.*

THE SHOWER OF LIGHT

This routine is designed to encourage you to open up to your feelings and improve communication.

1 *Stand in the starting position for the pump. With your arms at your sides, imagine a shower of light filling your entire body and spread your arms to a 45-degree angle with the palms facing up.*

2 *Slowly raise your arms upward until the elbows are about shoulder level, then bend them. Your hands should be about 15cm (6 in) from your head.*

3 *Press your arms downward in front of your body. When you get to just below the hips, begin again. Repeat the exercise about nine times to start, gradually building up to 20 repetitions in one session.*

THE PEBBLE IN THE LAKE

This exercise is designed to help you feel expanding energy all around you as you create a series of concentric circles. You should feel the expansion both back and front and attain a sense of space and personal freedom.

1 *Assume the starting position of the pump with your hands just in front of the lower abdomen. Reach forward with your arms, leading with the index fingers.*

2 *Move your hands to the sides of your body, palms down, imitating a ripple.*

3 *Concentrating on the insides of your hands, draw them back into the original position. Repeat at least nine times.*

135

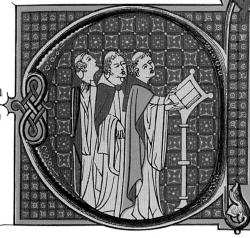

MEDIEVAL MONKS
Dr. Alfred Tomatis, a French physician and researcher in sound, claims that Gregorian chants are particularly therapeutic for the mind and body.

SHEN THERAPY

Shen therapy was devised by an American scientist, Richard Pavek, whose specialties were actually in electronics and chemistry. His analytical mind, however, led him to look for concrete evidence of the energy forces so often described in holistic therapies. He discovered that after any physical or emotional shock, the body tends to contract, forming a kind of spasm around the pain or perceived hurt. After a while the flow in this area may become so impaired that the removal of toxins is inhibited and the buildup of these toxins leads to tension and stress. Only by releasing the blockage with light, supportive touching can the symptoms be relieved

SOUND AND MUSIC THERAPIES

While children use their voices to shout anger or wail dismay, adults tend to repress these natural instincts and rarely use a fraction of their complete vocal range. Many therapists now believe that vocalizing our emotions can go a long way toward relieving stress. They suggest, for instance, that laughing and making other happy sounds when you feel depressed will lift your mood. As the breathing pattern automatically changes, the physiological and psychological states alter as well, increasing energy and boosting confidence. Some researchers believe that simply shouting or singing can help, while others identify particular sounds and behavior with emotional health. Alfred Tomatis, a French physician and researcher of sound, believes that the harmonic tones of Mozart and Gregorian chants have a neurophysiologic effect. He claims that the high frequency of these melodies stimulates the brain and nervous system and improves physical and mental functioning.

Other theorists believe that the body has its own resonant frequencies, which can vibrate out of harmony. Because particular parts of the body relate to different frequencies, determining the correct resonance of a dysfunctioning organ might help restore it. If a person suffers from liver problems, for

BIODANZA

Biodanza has roots in both therapy and dance. In 1960 Chilean Rolando Toro Araneda realized that Western dance had become very formalized and had lost much of the emotional expression of earlier tribal movement. He believed that we were denying our innate physical behavior and that if we were to dance in a manner true to our inner selves, we would release inhibition and literally dance our way to growth and wholeness.

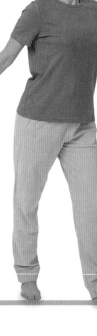

1 *Walk around the room, feeling your feet connected to the floor, and encourage your movements to become increasingly fluid.*

2 *Then put on some music that has a strong, fluid melody, and dance in any way that feels right, paying particular attention to your heart and chest.*

example, matching the liver with an appropriate sound vibration could help it return to its normal frequency and begin to heal itself. This rebalancing of the physical body should also aid relaxation and promote a general sense of equilibrium and harmony.

Singing can be therapeutic, but even if you think you can't sing, there are a number of sounds you can make in the privacy of your own home to help relieve stress. Humming is a good way to calm anxiety, and long elongated sighs can help reduce tension. Singing the different vowel sounds, such as *ooo, eeeeh,* and *uuuh,* can generally improve mood. It is important to forget convention when you make these sounds and just let yourself go. Focusing on where in your mouth and diaphragm the sounds are coming from can help you understand how they make you feel. Ultimately, just as a favorite piece of music can boost your mood and improve relaxation, so singing and humming can help to improve well-being.

For many years a number of health professionals have been including music therapy as part of their healing techniques. Music is often used to manage pain—for example, during surgery—and it may be incorporated into a rehabilitation program for someone who has a physical disability. Some psychotherapists have found that music is a good way to communicate with patients who cannot verbalize their problems. At the Rusk Institute for Rehabilitative Medicine in New York, music therapy has been integrated into programs for patients of all ages who have physical and/or mental disabilities.

DRAMA THERAPY

Like music, drama can provide an opportunity to loosen inhibitions. It allows a person to become immersed in another activity, to dismiss self-consciousness, and build a sense of self-worth. Drama therapy is especially effective in settings where individuals have difficulty relating to each other, for instance, in schools for emotionally disturbed children.

Much like the role play in gestalt therapy (see page 127), drama lets a person reenact specific situations and release unexpressed emotions. J. L. Moreno, who initially developed the concept of psychodrama, encouraged people in a group to play out each other's dilemmas. An unresolved family argument, for example, might be acted out with a different person adopting the role of each relative. The role of the key patient, or protagonist, is often played alternately by different members of the group. This helps everybody to see and attack the problem from different angles. While the therapist directs the scene according to what the protagonist reveals, the other members of the

continued on page 140

Transactional analysis
Drawing on humanistic beliefs, Eric Berne developed transactional analysis, a therapy that is designed to encourage and assert the uniqueness and fundamental healthiness of all individuals and help them control their own psychological destiny. In his popular book *I'm OK, You're OK,* Berne urged people to identify and dismantle the manipulative "games" and inappropriate "scripts" that hinder personal growth and consciously work toward self-healing.

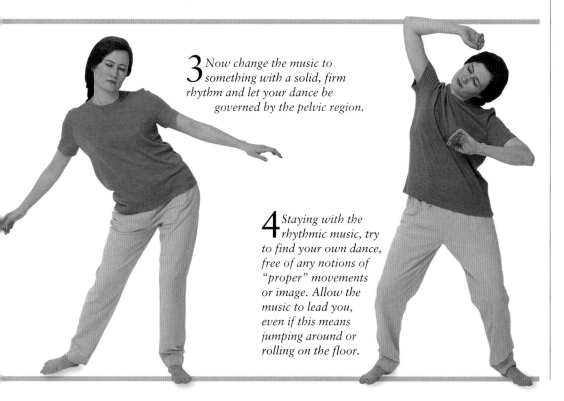

3 *Now change the music to something with a solid, firm rhythm and let your dance be governed by the pelvic region.*

4 *Staying with the rhythmic music, try to find your own dance, free of any notions of "proper" movements or image. Allow the music to lead you, even if this means jumping around or rolling on the floor.*

The Art Therapist

Art therapy is being used increasingly as a way to help people express feelings and release stress. Rather than attempting to paint or draw properly, patients are encouraged to abandon all expectations and simply see what happens.

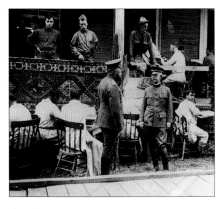

ART THERAPY
Soldiers traumatized during the First World War were sometimes encouraged to express their emotions and distress through painting.

VISUAL EXPRESSION
Art therapists usually offer a wide range of creative materials for patients to use to help release inhibition and express their inner emotional problems.

Art has been enjoyed as a means of relaxation since at least Egyptian times, but only since the early part of the 20th century has it been used as a systematic therapy. After the First World War many psychiatric patients were unable to communicate or articulate their feelings, and hospital art classes were used to encourage them to express their memories. As psychiatrists began to experiment with this therapy in treating other noncommunicative patients, they noticed the importance of visual expression for children. (See page 36 for more information on art

and children.) Further exploration has shown that art is an excellent way of releasing inhibition, providing young and old alike with the opportunity of free, unconscious expression. Contrary to some people's expectations, art therapy is not about learning to paint or draw with good technique. Instead, it prompts patients to forget their pre-conceptions and see what comes out.

Art therapists encourage patients to use a whole range of approaches—from painting and sketching to creating collages or sculpture—to express their emotions. The subject may be a theme, such as sleep or birth, selected by the therapist, or it may be one chosen by the client. Just as the creative process is thought to be therapeutic, so the final picture, no matter how incoherent it appears, can provide a source of contemplation and reflection.

The patient is encouraged to think about the images he or she has chosen and possibly even to speak to the picture, thinking about what it might say concerning its form and creator. When an object of fear is depicted, the emotion it elicits becomes objectified, releasing it from suppression and allowing it to exist in a physical form. The advantage of this approach is that a painting not only expresses emotions but can be physically put away, symbolically reinforcing an individual's ability to exert control over the subconscious. The confidence that this provides can then help the person to deal with other psychological issues.

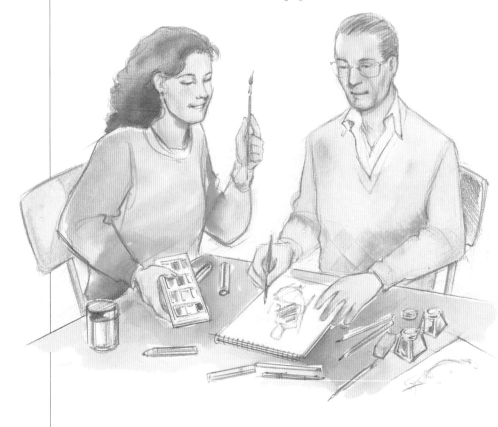

THE ROLE OF COLOR

Most people associate certain colors with particular moods or feelings. There is evidence to suggest, however, that color can actually play a therapeutic role—helping, for example, to improve calmness, provide inspiration, or increase energy. Yellow is associated with vibrancy and can aid in relieving gloom, while blue is related to cleansing and can help provide the inspiration to get rid of past anxieties and problems. Although many people associate red with anger, its energy can also be inspiring, and using this color for impulsive expressions of feeling may be beneficial. Pink is a warming color, while violet has a stimulating energy that some people believe suggests regeneration. Green's associations with nature provide a neutralizing, harmonious feeling. You might keep these different moods in mind when interpreting your own artwork.

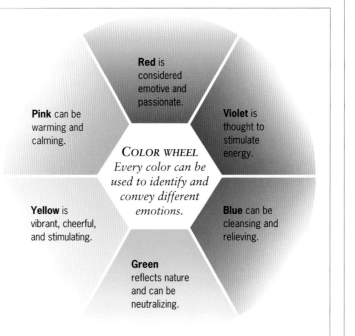

Red is considered emotive and passionate.

Pink can be warming and calming.

Violet is thought to stimulate energy.

COLOR WHEEL Every color can be used to identify and convey different emotions.

Yellow is vibrant, cheerful, and stimulating.

Blue can be cleansing and relieving.

Green reflects nature and can be neutralizing.

Where do art therapists work?

Art therapists work in a number of settings, from educational to hospital and prison facilities. Many specialize in working with children or geriatric patients. They may be called on to help identify emotional problems or to assist patients in coming to terms with particular difficulties.

What media do art therapists use?

Although painting is one of the main media used by art therapists, clients are usually invited to choose from a range of techniques. Drawing, painting, photography, sculpture, and metalwork can all be used as part of the self-healing process. Anything that encourages patients to express creativity and emotion is seen as a valuable means of therapy.

Do art therapists expect patients to be skilled in the therapeutic media?

Despite the initial skepticism of some clients, therapists do not expect any kind of skill in the art medium. Because art therapy is so subjective, it is impossible to make any mistakes or do anything wrong. In fact, nobody needs to understand the created image, other than the client. The essential insight of art therapy is that human expressive activity comes

in many forms, and as long as something has personal meaning, it will also have the potential to encourage individual growth. For this reason a client can produce what appears to be just a lot of colorful scribbling and yet still receive significant emotional and psychological benefit. The essence of art therapy is to find a subjective personal meaning in both the process and the final picture.

What are the professional requirements for an art therapist?

To qualify as a professional art therapist, a person must have completed a master's degree program approved by the American Art Therapy Association. Practitioners who meet the association's standards are given the title Art Therapist Registered (ATR) and are bound by the same code of confidentiality that applies to all psychotherapists.

WHAT YOU CAN DO AT HOME

Although working with a professional art therapist is more effective, you can still use artistic expression at home as a kind of self-help therapy. The only thing necessary is a willingness to give it a try. You could set yourself any theme, but the following exercise might be a good way to get started.

▶ *Draw, with as much detail as possible, a picture of how you would like to be.*

▶ *Draw, with as much detail as possible, a picture of how you see yourself now.*

▶ *Draw, with as much detail as possible, a picture of how you imagine someone that you love sees you.*

▶ *Consider the differences in the drawings. Try to write down in words what the differences are.*

▶ *Consider the differences among the three drawings that you are unable to describe easily.*

▶ *Try to classify or comment on the aspects of the drawings that seem to sit outside language. It may be that they point toward an area in your inner emotional life that would benefit from further personal reflection. You could simply contemplate these aspects, thinking about how they fit into the way you envision your personal growth, or use them in subsequent consultations with a therapist.*

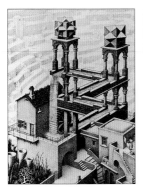

ABSORBING ARTWORK
Focusing on a picture that has lots of intriguing detail, such as this one by 20th-century graphic artist Maurits C. Escher, can help you lose yourself in contemplation.

group try to identify with the different scenarios. After a session, everybody sits down to discuss what they felt and how they interpreted the situation.

Drama therapy is effective because it allows individuals to focus vividly on a situation that needs resolving and play it out in a nonthreatening situation. By assuming a dramatic role, many people can act out pent-up emotions they might not be able to express otherwise.

RELAXATION

Setting aside quiet time for yourself and creating a comfortable environment in which to enjoy it are important first steps to improving your relaxation abilities. Taking time off on a regular basis will help you not only to cope better with the tribulations of daily life but also to maintain the emotional balance needed for good mental health.

Creating the right environment

Don't plan to try to unwind if you know that there could be an imminent phone call or visitor at the door. Instead, try to choose a period—even if it's only 15 minutes—in which you know that you can relax uninterrupted. If possible, choose an area away from the usual distractions. For example, if you work at home, use a room other than your office or studio so that you can feel both physically and emotionally separated from work pressures. A serene setting with

soft lighting and pleasant visual images will help you get into a calmer frame of mind, as will some gentle background music.

If you find it hard to forget your self-consciousness, try focusing on an interesting picture to help you lose all immediate awareness. A busy picture is particularly good because you must gradually increase your concentration to interpret and absorb all that is going on. Anything that helps you to become absorbed in something other than your immediate troubles and anxieties will help you relax. While some people may choose to use traditional meditation or visualization techniques as part of their relaxation time, others gain as much benefit from sitting in contemplation using their own individual approach.

Aromatherapy can be used to enhance the relaxing atmosphere of your chosen area. A few drops of essential oil on a pillow, for example, or some aromatic candles will help to set the right mood for a little self-indulgence and relaxation. If you find your most pleasurable moments are those spent in the bath, a few drops of aromatherapy oil added to the bathwater will improve your sense of tranquillity even more. Essential oils can also be added to a carrier oil and used for a relaxing massage—either given by a professional or a partner. You can experiment with different oils to find out which ones enhance your frame of mind (see box below for suggestions).

RELAXING WITH AROMATHERAPY

There are a number of essential plant oils that can be used for relaxation. While some target specific problems, such as anxiety, others help to promote a general sense of calmness and well-being. Many people find that adding a few drops of oil to bathwater or placing a little oil in a vaporizer can be effective. Even aromatic

candles can help to create the right environment for relaxation. Always check an oil for specific health warnings or contraindications because some must be avoided in certain circumstances, such as pregnancy. If you plan to use oil directly on the skin, mix it first with a carrier oil, such as almond or grapeseed.

OIL	USE
Chamomile	A particularly soothing oil, chamomile reduces restlessness and worry.
Lavender	A good oil for relieving fear and anxiety, lavender induces relaxation.
Marjoram	With its warming qualities, marjoram improves circulation and calmness.
Neroli	Particularly fragrant, neroli is associated with relief of stress and shock.
Jasmine	Luxurious in aroma, jasmine can relieve depression and fear.

CHAPTER 7

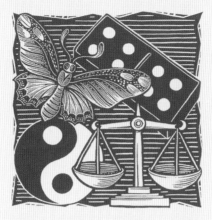

MAINTAINING MENTAL BALANCE

---

*The essence of emotional health and
happiness lies in finding a sense of personal
equilibrium. This chapter explores some of the
simple steps you can take toward improving your
general lifestyle and outlook and achieving
greater balance in your emotions.*

STAYING ON AN EVEN KEEL

When you are emotionally balanced, you feel in control of your life. Realistic expectations and a calm approach to living can help you realize inner peace and long-lasting contentment.

In everybody's life there are periods of joy as well as of difficulty or sadness. The emotions you experience at such times can distort your view of life, making you unrealistically optimistic or unnecessarily pessimistic. To remain on an even keel during highs and lows, you need to maintain a rational perspective, not getting too carried away by the good times or feeling too bitterly disappointed during the bad.

No matter what your current experiences are, it is important to remember that all kinds of feelings come and go; excitement has to fade and bad times generally do get better. Keeping all these things in mind can be difficult. We all overreact on occasion, becoming emotionally overwrought as circumstances sweep over us and we find it increasingly difficult to maintain control. Nevertheless, by seeking a balance and by constantly aiming to be healthy and happy, we can live fulfilling and satisfying lives most of the time.

FINDING HAPPINESS

Despite the common conceptions that having a little more money or perhaps a busier social life would make us happier, research suggests that we have a basic level of contentedness to which we tend to return, despite disruptions in our usual lifestyle. An American study conducted in 1975 by the *Journal of Personality and Social Psychology* followed the lives of individuals who had won large sums of money in the Illinois State Lottery and, at the same time, of other people who had been severely paralyzed in accidents. As might be expected, the happiness of the lottery winners increased greatly at first and that of the accident victims fell sharply. But over the following months, both sets of people reported that their happiness levels were gradually returning to normal. The two groups were adapting to the changes in their lives and adjusting their expectations about what life had to offer them in the future.

The evidence suggests that most people have a fairly constant level of happiness throughout life, regardless of such factors as social status, race, income, or education. The element that appears to be most important in influencing happiness is personality. Our personal style, whether it is outgoing or reserved, cheerful or stolid, will affect our objectives in life, encouraging us to seek the company or relative solitude that we desire. This basic level of happiness will be overlaid occasionally with spells of intense joy or sadness, but most people adjust appropriately to changing circumstances and return eventually to their "normal" state.

Expectations also play a major role in determining your basic level of happiness by setting up a difference between what you expect from life and what you actually have. As your circumstances change, you increase or decrease your expectations accordingly. For example, you might have a reasonably comfortable life on your current income but you might also believe that you would be happier if you were earning twice your present salary. If your income were to double tomorrow, however, you would probably soon get used to spending the extra money and eventually start thinking how much better life would be if only you could double your income once again.

AN EVEN KEEL
Psychiatrist Carl Jung once claimed that the sea is a symbol for the emotions. This is reflected in common sayings such as "jumping in at the deep end," "turning with the tide," and "maintaining an even keel."

BUDDHIST VISUALIZATION

The word *metta* describes a feeling of loving kindness and concern for the well-being of other people. It is a spontaneous expression of a desire to help and is based on communal awareness of human-kind. Metta is unrelated to a person's attraction or love for another; it is simply a reflection of concern for people in general, regardless of specific reasons or situations. Cultivating feelings of warmth for others also helps improve your own self-perception and emotional well-being. The following meditation, often used to visualize and express this Buddhist concept, aims to increase sensations of inner peace and generosity.

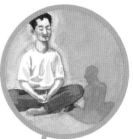

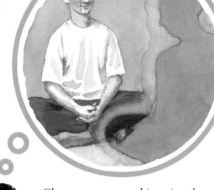

Close your eyes and imagine that a person of infinite kindness and love is sitting opposite you. Your hearts are linked by some force—perhaps a golden light—and as you breathe in, you absorb this goodness.

Feel the figure opposite you gradually diminishing in size as you become increasingly strong and full of love. Although the person is always there as a source of wisdom, you are now able to provide a healing, calming energy as well.

Now imagine someone who is in trouble and distress and connect your heart with that person's. As you breathe in, absorb some of his or her troubles, and as you breathe out, pass on some of your love and strength. Feel the positive sense of balance and self-awareness as you offer support.

Balance and moderation

Long-term contentment and inner peace stem from having realistic expectations. Accepting the realities of life and taking its ups and downs in stride provide a good rational basis for aspirations.

A central theme for happiness in many philosophies is the concept of balance. Plato described "the golden mean" as being the most positive course of action and behavior. He proposed that an individual should always take the middle path and enjoy "all things in moderation."

Finding the middle path through self-reflection and contemplation underpins many Eastern approaches to life, including Zen Buddhism and Taoism. One route to such enlightenment is the ancient practice of meditation, which can be used by anybody to improve personal happiness.

The relatively new Western practice of Neuro Linguistic Programming also advocates reflection and self-awareness as ways to reach one's full potential. It encourages individuals to become more flexible in their thinking, asserting that they can benefit from examining and adjusting their attitudes to achieve greater happiness. If a person finds life to be unfulfilling, NLP proposes that it may be necessary to consider the possibility that his or her actions are inappropriate.

ZEN BUDDHISM

In recent years increasing numbers of Westerners have turned to Zen Buddhism to help them make sense of life and cope with its difficulties. The principal aim of Zen is the attainment of spiritual enlightenment—a sense of inner peace, balance, and mind-fulness. It is based on a series of beliefs and actions that are thought to be essentially "right" and that promote both personal and emotional development.

The Middle Way

In Zen, as in all Buddhist teaching, the route of moderation is known as the Middle Way or Noble Eightfold Path. The first step on this path is to cultivate rightness, or perfect understanding, by learning not to be too opinionated or hold rigid views and by seeing life realistically, without undue optimism or pessimism. This step also involves discarding negative emotions, such as greed, self-delusion, pride, hate, and doubt.

The second step is to strive for perfect emotion; it refers to the attitude, or frame of mind, with which you approach daily life. It stresses cultivating more positive emotions, such as love and joy, and yet encourages you to be less idealistic. This step helps individuals to understand the origins and consequences of their thoughts by facing them and seeking equanimity.

The third step is to achieve perfect speech, which, in essence, means being truthful. By choosing words carefully and exercising self-restraint, a person can enjoy a sense of open honesty in relationships that will make them more satisfying. The aim is to maintain harmony by pursuing openness and at the same time avoiding momentary pleasure at the expense of somebody else.

The fourth step is perfect action, which involves behaving in a reasonable manner that is appropriate to the situation. By inviting a person to analyze his or her actions and motivation, this step encourages self-awareness, which is particularly important in achieving mental balance. The fifth step,

> **DID YOU KNOW?**
> Many people think that meditation requires total emptiness of the mind. In reality, however, hearing heavy traffic going past or considering what to have for dinner need not destroy your meditative process, providing that it does not cause inattention. Allow such interruptions to come and go, accepting and noticing their presence but avoiding judgment or elaboration.

perfect livelihood, entails finding the most suitable way to earn a living and is closely related to the sixth step—perfect effort. This is the good work that you will be capable of when patience and persistence have helped you to master the tribulations of existence.

The seventh step, perfect awareness, relates to the development of mental tranquillity. It encourages acknowledgment of the self and of all forms and existences that surround us. This, together with the eighth concept, perfect *Samadhi*, or completeness, can help individuals to focus their thoughts. Promoting a clear and open state, the eighth step encourages understanding beyond ordinary consciousness, developing a sense of "perfect absorption." Each step depends on all the others to enable complete mental harmony and concerted application.

THE NOBLE EIGHTFOLD PATH

Buddhism teaches a series of eight steps that will eventually lead to personal and spiritual completeness. Providing both spiritual and practical guidance, the stages encourage full emotional development and acceptance of life, which can help individuals come to a better understanding of both themselves and others. By thinking, acting, speaking, and living in the "correct" way, followers should find a sense of balance, improving both their personal and social happiness. Essentially, Zen Buddhist practitioners believe in moderation in all things and that only through meditating and cultivating the correct way to live can we achieve true enlightenment.

THE PATH TO ENLIGHTENMENT
Each step of the Noble Eightfold Path takes an individual nearer to enlightenment. All actions and qualities work together to provide a sense of balance and harmony.

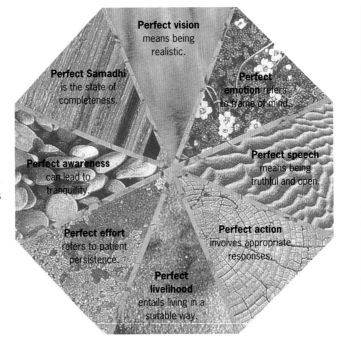

Perfect vision means being realistic.

Perfect Samadhi is the state of completeness.

Perfect emotion refers to frame of mind.

Perfect awareness can lead to tranquillity.

Perfect speech means being truthful and open.

Perfect effort refers to patient persistence.

Perfect action involves appropriate responses.

Perfect livelihood entails living in a suitable way.

TAOISM

Taoism, the way or the path, is an ancient Chinese philosophy that underpins much of traditional Chinese medicine. Like Zen Buddhism, it aims to help its followers achieve inner peace and live in harmony with the world around them. It is based on the belief that everything exists through the interaction of two forces, or energies, known as *yin* and *yang*. For life to be in harmony, yin, the universal feminine force, must be in balance with yang, the universal masculine force.

In addition to yin and yang, which permeate both the animate and the inanimate, Taoist theory identifies three elements that are essential to life. These elements, known as the Three Treasures, bring health, happiness, and longevity when balanced correctly. The first treasure, *jing,* represents vital essence and the physical body; the second, *chi,* relates to life energy; the third, *shen* embodies spirit, which includes the soul, thoughts, and emotions.

Taoists believe that a balance of these essences and life forces can be attained only through correct diet, exercise, and outlook. Whereas most people allow external stimuli to affect their energy, Taoists try to use their minds to master it. By attempting to direct and harness the life force in every physical and emotional aspect, Taoists aim to achieve a complete sense of balance. They believe that disease and degeneration occur when we fail to follow an appropriate lifestyle. A failing immune system, for example, might result from an unsuitable diet, and it may also reflect a negative outlook. By looking

Origins

It is believed that the ideas of Taoism have existed for 6,000 years or more and were first handed down by oral tradition. Many of its teachings come from Lao-tzu, who may have lived in the 6th century B.C., though it is still debated whether he is a historical or legendary figure. The first known written record of Taoist principles is the *Tao Te Ching* ("The Way and Its Power"), dating from the 3rd or 4th century B.C. Based on Lao-tzu's work, it provides followers with both practical guidance and philosophical theory.

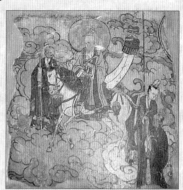

LAO-TZU
Pictured here on horseback, Lao-tzu is the ancient Chinese sage credited with devising the principles of Taoism.

after your spiritual and physical life forces, you are working with nature and resisting ill health and anxiety. This empathy with nature involves accepting and moving with change. Flexibility and receptiveness are key elements of Taoist good health.

The Taoist sage Lao-tzu taught that it is counterproductive to try to shape the flow of events by going against the natural order of things. The way to master circumstances is to understand their nature and then shape your actions in accordance with these principles. The physical expression of this idea is found in the flowing, meditative movements of the exercise t'ai chi ch'uan.

YIN AND YANG FOODS

According to Chinese philosophy, foods are divided into yin and yang categories. Yin foods have cool, calming qualities; yang foods are warm and stimulating. It is therefore possible to choose foods so that they help shape your energies and control excessive emotional tendencies. The samples below are typical.

YIN FOODS	YANG FOODS	YIN FOODS	YANG FOODS
Boiled foods	Fried foods	Some fish	Shellfish
Salad greens	Onions, garlic	Potatoes	Beef
Milk	Eggs	Duck	Chicken
Winter squash	Eggplant, tomatoes	Tofu, bean sprouts	Peanuts
Melons, pears	Tangerines, persimmons	Honey	Vinegar

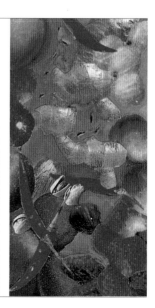

The Zen Teacher

The basis of Zen is a search for inner peace. In achieving an internal sense of calm and balance, you learn to accept and enjoy life as it really is instead of making yourself unhappy by constantly striving for impossible goals.

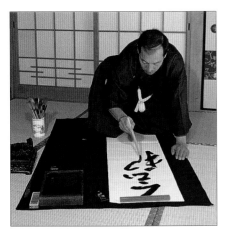

CALLIGRAPHY
Some Zen teachers and followers practice the art of calligraphy in order to improve their inner balance and tranquillity.

At the heart of Zen is the attempt to perceive the true nature of existence. This involves learning to see the essential nature of yourself and of everything around you. By realizing that there is no division between yourself and the rest of the universe and that you are an integral part of life, you also learn that there is nothing to fear. This enlightenment is achieved through meditation (*za-zen*), the guidance of a Zen teacher (*roshi*), membership in a Zen association or community (*sangha*), and studying the teachings of Buddha (*Dharma*). It makes use of concepts like sparseness, control, and spontaneity to reach total understanding.

Origins

Zen, as it is known in Japan and the West, and *Cha'an,* as it is called in China, is based in part on the teachings of Bodhi-dharma, a Buddhist monk who carried Buddhism from India to China in about A.D. 520. In its early years there, Zen was greatly influenced by the Chinese philosophy of Taoism, and many of its elements, such as chanting rituals and nonverbal teaching, bear a strong resemblance to Taoist practices. From China, Zen spread to Korea and then in the 12th century to Japan, where it still has most of its strongest links.

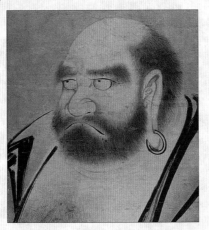

BODHIDHARMA
Bodhidharma, the traveling Indian monk, is credited with taking Zen teachings and practices to China.

The Four Noble Truths
The core of Buddhist teaching is contained within the "Four Noble Truths," which diagnose and aim to reconcile the different aspects of human suffering. The first of these, discontent, or suffering, is known as *dukkha;* it reflects the natural and inevitable pains of birth, aging, grief, and sorrow. The second aspect asserts that life itself is experienced as suffering because we react with negative expectations and emotions. Greed, for example, which reflects the impulse to grab what we want; hatred, the desire to push away what we dislike; and ignorance, in which we try to hide ourselves from problems, are all responses with which we commonly approach life.

The third Noble Truth involves learning to accept life as it is, following the Noble Eightfold Path (see page 144) and seeking moderation in all thoughts and actions. The fourth Noble Truth encourages the follower to focus on the role that thoughts have in sustaining illusions about the self.

Practicing Zen
While Zen Buddhism does not have any ritualistic doctrines, it does encourage specific behaviors that promote personal development and fulfillment. Cultivating meditation techniques, for instance, and seeking to improve one's outlook and sense of tranquillity require a certain amount of individual commitment. Buddhism is a nontheistic religion, however, which means that it does

ZEN CLASSES
Zen teachers help their students to practice meditation skills and chanting. They also read Zen scriptures occasionally.

not require its followers to believe in a god or gods. While most people can learn a lot about the concepts of Zen by reading and studying the teachings of Buddha, it can also be useful to get the help of a Zen teacher, who will assist with meditation techniques. The basic principles of Zen practice are easy to grasp, but appreciating its subtleties and acquiring the wisdom and understanding that Zen can bring require perseverance and dedication. The art of Zen and its potential path to enlightenment is an ongoing, essentially lifelong experience, and its practitioners never actually stop learning or working to improve their skills.

What is Zen training like?

Most Zen training follows one of the two Japanese schools: Soto and Rinzai. While both of them focus on the importance of meditation, Soto is known as the gradual path and Rinzai tends to emphasize the dramatic. Both stress the effort and thinking needed to attain enlightenment, but Rinzai uses a stricter training approach that insists on meditators perfecting their posture and ability to concentrate.

All schools that follow the Rinzai tradition and some that follow the Soto version of Zen make extensive use of *koans*, which are traditional, paradoxical stories (riddles) that the teacher gives the students to solve. Many schools also require study of Buddhist teachings and chanting. One of the main focuses of the teaching, however, is to encourage individuals to learn how to sit in contemplation. By focusing on the self in the current moment and accepting all that such existence entails, students gradually learn how Zen can lead to insight.

Most people who learn Zen from a teacher will study mainly meditation techniques. Only when they have mastered these skills sufficiently can they progress to a more rigorous study of Buddhist philosophy.

How long does a session last?

A Zen session may go on for a couple of hours or more. It is usually divided into periods of seated meditation, each one lasting from 20 to 50 minutes, which are separated by short periods of walking meditation, or *kinhin*.

Some people go on Zen meditation retreats (*sesshin*), which typically last about a week but may involve just a weekend. Each day is structured to include fixed periods of meditation, reading from Buddhist texts, and chanting of Zen vows.

WHAT YOU CAN DO AT HOME

Advanced Zen meditation requires studying with a master, but you can practice a basic technique on your own. All you have to do is sit in a comfortable position for about 20 minutes and focus your mind on the rhythm of your breathing.

Begin by sitting comfortably on a chair or cross-legged on the floor, with your neck and spine straight and upright. Let your shoulders relax and place your hands in your lap, palms upward. Half-close your eyes and focus them on the floor in front of you. Allow your breathing to continue naturally at its own rhythm and start to count your breaths: count 1 on your first inhalation, 2 when you exhale, 3 when you inhale again, and so on. The aim is to reach a count of 10 without being distracted by any intrusive thoughts. If you do get distracted, go back to 1 and start again. When you reach 10, return to 1 and keep repeating the process for 20 minutes.

Zen Garden

A Zen garden is a place of quiet and serenity, a space designed to encourage contemplation and meditation, where you can let your mind relax and escape from the pressures of the outside world.

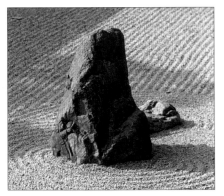

GARDEN OF CONTEMPLATION
Rock formations surrounded by carefully patterned sand or stones provide a peaceful place in which to sit and engage in quiet contemplation.

Many practitioners of Zen create special garden landscapes, known as *karesansui*, to aid contemplation. Coarse gravel or small stones raked in rippled patterns are used to symbolize the sea, a lake, or a river. A few rocks or stones are then set like islands in the gravel.

The Zen gardens designed and built in Japan by Zen priests and monks contain subtly symbolic elements of the Zen tradition. A single rock standing in an expanse of gravel, for instance, might symbolize a single thought that is surrounded by the infinity of the universe. Or if circular ripples are raked into the gravel around a rock, the garden may represent the way that thought distorts the pure experience of reality.

You do not need to understand its symbolism to benefit from the calm, meditative state that a Zen garden inspires. And it is easy to create your own version for peaceful reflection.

CREATING A SIMPLE ZEN GARDEN

To make your own Zen garden, first clear the vegetation from a roughly rectangular piece of ground of whatever size you choose or can manage. If possible, this piece of ground should have a plain backdrop—to prevent distraction—and be edged with stones or wooden boards to neatly contain the gravel. At one or more points in the area, place a small rock, sunk about one-third into the ground.

When your rock or rocks are in place, cover the ground with a reasonable depth of coarse gravel or pebbles, preferably off-white or gray, then use a wide wooden rake to create a circular pattern of ripples around each rock and a pattern of straight ripples running parallel to the longer sides of the garden. You can rework or alter the pattern whenever you choose.

If you do not have access to outdoor space, you can create a smaller version in a tray, using sand with one or two beautiful stones placed in it. You can trace your designs or ripples with your fingers or a small, sharp stick. The tray can be kept on a windowsill, shelf, or table, or wherever it is convenient for you to sit quietly and contemplate.

YOUR OWN ZEN GARDEN
Once the basic garden has been set up, you can rearrange your stones and gravel as many times as you wish. Take care not to make the garden too active or varied, however, as the effect could become distracting during contemplation.

MAINTAINING A
POSITIVE OUTLOOK

Having an optimistic outlook in life will help you feel more contented. If you look ahead constructively and keep a sense of humor, problems are less likely to get you down.

One secret of achieving mental balance is to maintain an affirmative outlook, trying always to think positively about yourself and life in general. It is important to make positive thinking an integral part of your outlook and behavior, even if this takes a certain amount of conscious effort. By overcoming any tendency toward cynicism or pessimism, you can eventually train yourself to be affirming and outgoing and to believe firmly in yourself and your own capabilities.

Emile Coué, a French pharmacist turned psychotherapist, was one of the first people of the modern era to promote positive thinking. He opened a free psychotherapy clinic in Nancy, France, in 1910, where he encouraged his clients to empty their minds of negative thoughts and replace them with positive ones. He believed that by doing this, they could train their subconscious minds to be more positive. He recommended that they repeat the phrase "Every day, in every way, I am getting better and better"

DAILY AFFIRMATIONS

Affirmations are short statements that express a positive belief in yourself. Used on a daily basis, they are a simple but effective way of giving yourself encouragement and reassurance and building lasting self-confidence.

If you are going through a difficult period or simply feel a need to be more positive about yourself, choose or write down a new affirmation for each day. The best ones are short, simple, and focused on a single theme or subject. Statements that are complicated or are aimed at more than one target will lose their impact and be more difficult to remember. It is important, though, not to concentrate so much on the wording that you lose sight of the message. Write and recall your thoughts in the present tense, which will help you to affirm that the possibility already exists, rather than stating a hope for the future. For instance, instead of writing "I am going to enjoy my job," say "I enjoy my job." Always make the statement completely

positive. "I am successful" is far better than "I am not a failure." You can create affirmations to help you be more positive about your personality ("I have a good sense of humor"), your abilities ("I am good at my job"), your relationships with other people ("I have many friends"), and any other area of your life that you want to improve. In fact, the greater the spectrum of affirmations, the more complete your sense of self should become. In the morning, look in the mirror and say an affirmation out loud to yourself, then keep it in your mind throughout the day so that it seeps into your subconscious. Repeat it whenever you feel negative or stressed. If you begin to doubt your abilities at any time, take a deep breath and recall your statements.

SELF-AFFIRMATION
Always keeping your affirmations close at hand will help you to gain the confidence and self-belief you need to face the tribulations of daily life.

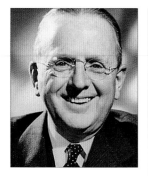

NORMAN VINCENT PEALE (1898–1993) Minister at the Marble Collegiate Church in New York City for 52 years, Peale popularized the benefits of constructive thought with his book The Power of Positive Thinking, *published in 1952.*

to speed up the process. Research by American psychologists more than 50 years later showed that such simple statements are, in fact, effective. The public seemed to agree. Some 20 million copies in 41 languages of Norman Vincent Peale's book *The Power of Positive Thinking* have been sold since it was first published in 1952.

A GUIDE TO POSITIVE THINKING

The theory behind positive thinking is that by learning to reject negative tendencies, you become happier and healthier and better able to cope with life's difficulties. Many psychological studies have lent support to this concept by showing how the mind can influence our emotions and health (see pages 16–19 and pages 28–30).

The best way to develop the habit of positive thinking is to build it one day at a time. Beginning the day in a good frame of mind is particularly important; start the morning with a resolution that things are going to go well. As the day progresses, use constructive thinking to avoid creating difficulties or imagining problems where none exist. By approaching tasks and events with a determination to succeed, many people find that chores become much easier. For example, it

doesn't pay to avoid difficult or boring jobs simply because you are not looking forward to doing them. Postponement leads only to further anxiety and stress, so it becomes difficult to relax and even more wearisome to get on with them.

The best way to deal with unappealing tasks is to tackle them at the earliest possible opportunity so that they are out of the way and you can enjoy the rest of the day. And when you encounter any problems at work or in your personal life, look at them as obstacles that you can and will overcome by figuring out solutions or the best way to cope with their consequences. When something goes wrong, concentrate on finding the best way forward rather than brooding about what has happened.

Thinking positively can also improve your relationships with other people. At its simplest, this means accepting that everyone, yourself included, has characteristics or habits that others find irritating but they also have many good and likable qualities. If you learn to recognize and change your own bad habits, your good side will become more apparent and people will respond to it. Similarly, if you are tolerant of the weaknesses of others and pay attention to

DEVELOPING CONFIDENCE

There are certain moments and events in life that can make it more difficult than usual to think positively about yourself. Important meetings or interviews, for example, can cause a lot of anxiety and worry. A buildup of excessive tension or nervousness may then undermine your self-esteem and affect your performance. Imagining yourself in the situation beforehand can be a valuable way of becoming mentally prepared. By stimulating the range of emotions that you are likely to feel, you can learn to recognize and overcome the areas in which you lack confidence or feel negative. This practice should help you feel better when facing the forthcoming event and enable you to do your best.

Picture yourself at the beginning of the interview, incorporating all the details you can remember from similar experiences. Expect to feel anxious but be positive in your attitude.

Run through the whole meeting in your mind, anticipating the questions you are likely to be asked and how you will answer them. Consider your performance as you go. How do you feel about the way you are presenting yourself?

their better qualities, you will come to enjoy their company more. Try not to be intimidated by other people or their abilities because even if they appear to be always in control and self-confident, they probably have their own feelings of insecurity and self-doubt to wrestle with at times.

Believe in your own skills and talents, and if somebody criticizes you, don't give in to negative feelings of hurt or anger. Instead, think about what was said and why. If the criticism was unjustified or simply spiteful, either let it pass or tactfully explain to the person who made it why he or she was mistaken. If it was justified, take it as an opportunity to learn from your mistakes so that you can avoid repeating them.

Throughout the day, if negative feelings, doubts, or anxieties about a situation enter your mind, replace them with thoughts of coping and succeeding. Sometimes negative feelings are not very specific but take the form of a more general sense of gloom. To prevent such negativity from feeding upon itself and becoming self-perpetuating, cancel it out by replacing it with positive, optimistic thoughts about the good things in life—such as your favorite music, movies, people, or places—or by making plans for

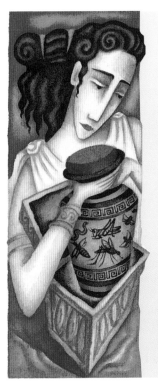

Fables and behavior

PANDORA'S BOX

The term *Pandora's box* comes from an ancient Greek legend. As the story goes, the powerful god Zeus arranged for the creation of a beautiful woman—Pandora—who would be sent to release evil into the world as punishment of Prometheus for creating and helping man. She arrived with a box in which was enclosed a jar containing every kind of evil. When the box was opened, all of these evils flew out and have afflicted humankind ever since. However, the box also contained the gift of hope, which remains as an appropriate symbol of the quintessential importance of a positive attitude in overcoming the tribulations of life.

something to look forward to. Essentially, positive thinking is about focusing on the good that you and the world have to offer each other and believing in your ability to make things even better.

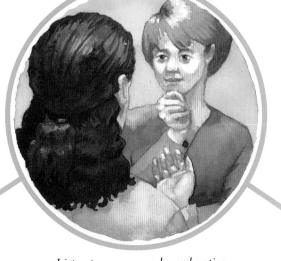

Listen to your remarks and notice the effect they are having. Picture people listening attentively to your comments; they want to hear what you are saying. If you feel any doubts or anxieties about the way you are responding, push them away and keep calm and focused.

When you feel comfortable with your performance, play the image back in your mind like a rehearsal. By relating to those attitudes that made you feel calm and in control, you should start to feel confident with the situation and better able to deal with the real interview when it happens.

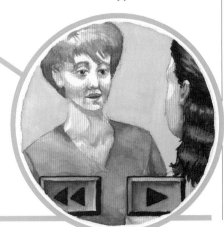

Dealing with Life's Ups and Downs

To feel good mentally, you also need to feel fit and healthy physically. Good diet, regular exercise and relaxation, and adequate rest are all necessary for emotional well-being.

The mind and body influence each other in numerous ways. When you feel happy and content, you are less likely to suffer from minor ailments. Similarly, if you are fit and healthy, it is easier to have a happy and positive outlook. A body that is unwell or not functioning at its full capacity does not provide a good basis for coping with the realities of daily life. One of the keys to happiness is maintaining good physical and emotional health. Working to keep yourself in shape means acknowledging the importance that healthy living can have on your emotional well-being. If you have one aspect of good health, you will more likely have the other.

KEEP IN SHAPE

To keep yourself in good physical shape, you need a healthy diet and enough exercise to maintain a good level of fitness. A healthy diet is one that provides the balance of nutrients and raw materials that your body needs for energy and for maintaining

---

REDUCING STRESS WITH TAOIST EXERCISE

Taoists believe that nurturing life and maintaining balance involves staying as flexible as possible. Special exercises help to keep essential fluids and vital energy flowing freely and encourage internal focus and full self-control. Through deep, controlled breathing and rhythmic physical movement, the body and breathing of an individual are harmonized and vital energy is circulated to every tissue and organ. These activities, which promote mental and physical relaxation, contrast with many Western exercises, which rely on extreme exertion to produce any effect.

Taoist exercises should be performed just before going to bed. They will relax the muscles, make you feel calm, and help you to enjoy a good night's sleep.

1 SPINE AND TORSO TWIST
Stand with your legs shoulder width apart; raise your right arm to shoulder height and rest your left hand on your hip. Moving the thighs only, twist your torso slowly to the left, hold for a second, and then return to the original position. Do 30 to 50 twists one way and then the other.

Keep the feet firmly positioned as you twist the torso.

2 BUMP AND GRIND Stand *facing forward with your feet shoulder width apart. Let your weight rest on your thighs with your knees slightly bent. Raise your arms above your head, then rotate your hips and pelvis in large circles, as though you were swinging a hula hoop. Perform the exercise 10 to 12 times in each direction.*

Knees should be slightly bent as the body rotates.

and repairing itself. Depending on their levels of physical activity, average adults need between 6 and 11 servings of carbohydrate-rich foods, such as bread, pasta, and rice, every day and at least 5 servings of fresh fruits and vegetables. They should also eat 2 to 3 servings each of dairy products and protein-rich foods such as lean meat, fish, poultry, beans, peas, and lentils.

Regular exercise is vitally important for the body because it helps the organs and muscles function more efficiently, improves circulation, and makes you less prone to illness. It also speeds up your metabolism, strengthens your bones, and helps to reduce stress, a factor that can increase blood pressure and lead to heart disease and stroke. For basic good fitness, all you need is about half an hour a day of moderate exercise; this can be any physical activity that makes you feel slightly out of breath. Brisk walking is an inexpensive and easy way to get this kind of exercise; so, too, are activities like cycling and swimming. You can incorporate moderate exercise into your daily routine in many ways: for example, using the stairs instead of an elevator and walking all or part of the way to work or the store instead of driving or using public transportation.

REGULAR RELAXATION

One of the best ways to help yourself cope with the physical and emotional stresses of everyday life is to set aside time for relaxation. Some people use meditation techniques (see page 113), but simply sitting still and clearing your mind can also be effective. It's useful to do some kind of relaxation exercise every day, more often if you feel under intense pressure or anxiety.

There are many different ways to relax; some are more effective than others, but anything that helps you to unwind can be

WARNING

If you want to do strenuous forms of exercise, such as aerobics, working out in a gym, or playing an energetic sport like squash, have a medical checkup first to make sure that you don't have any disorder that could make such exertion dangerous.

A TAOIST RECIPE FOR SHRIMP

Taoists believe there is an intrinsic link between the health of the body and the mind and have devised dietary approaches to promote well-being. The following recipe contains garlic, which boosts the immune system and helps lower blood pressure and cholesterol levels. It also includes ginger and chilies, which aid digestion and circulation and may also prevent blood clots that can lead to heart attack and stroke.

120 ml/4 fl oz soy sauce
175 ml/6 fl oz rice wine
3 tbsp sugar
900 g/2 lb large shrimp
3–4 tbsp cooking oil
5–6 cloves garlic
2 green onions
5-cm/2-in piece fresh ginger
55 g/2 oz red chilies

- In a large bowl, stir together the soy sauce, rice wine, and sugar.
- Shell and devein the shrimp and add them to the marinade, coating them thoroughly; marinate for 15 minutes. Drain but reserve the marinade.
- Finely chop the garlic, green onions, ginger, and chilies; mix together. Divide the mixture into two equal portions.
- Heat the oil in a wok over medium heat. Add half of the garlic mixture and cook until the garlic turns golden.
- Raise the heat to high, add the shrimp and cook for 2 to 3 minutes. Add the remaining garlic mixture and stir-fry for 3 minutes.
- Add the marinade and a little more soy sauce and wine if you wish. Lower the heat to medium and simmer for 5 minutes.

Serves 4

helpful. If you just need to take your mind off your problems, try simple leisure activities, such as listening to music, reading, going for a walk, spending time on a hobby or other interest, or sitting quietly and putting your mind into neutral.

For deeper relaxation, especially when you are feeling very stressed or anxious, try more direct methods that have an almost immediate calming effect on your mind and body. The more advanced of these, such as yoga and transcendental meditation, require some training and practice, but simple deep-breathing exercises and muscle relaxation routines can also be very effective.

When you relax, your heart rate and blood pressure drop, muscle tension eases, and the flow of blood to your skin and vital organs increases. These effects not only

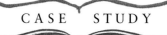
An Eczema Sufferer

Mental and emotional stress can be expressed in different ways. Physical symptoms ranging from coughs and colds to headaches and back pain are common, as are skin conditions, which can often worsen during periods of acute anxiety. Curing the illness is as much about addressing the underlying cause as it is about attacking the symptoms.

Alan is 38 and works as a sales representative for a computer and technical equipment company. Falling profit margins have recently led to a cut in the size of his sales force, and Alan now has to cover larger areas and meet higher targets. As a result, he finds himself sometimes working 12-hour days, often skipping lunch, and getting home late and too tired to bother eating properly. As he was driving home one recent evening, he noticed that the backs of his knees and the insides of his elbows felt itchy. The next day he could see that these areas were very red and inflamed. Despite the use of a cream, the condition has been getting increasingly worse, and Alan's doctor has diagnosed stress-related eczema.

WHAT SHOULD ALAN DO?

Although Alan suffered from eczema once before as a young child, he has been free of it until now. His doctor has prescribed a mild hydrocortisone cream to treat the itching from the eczema, but this will not address the stress that triggered the problem. Unless Alan can find some way of changing his working conditions, there is a good chance that the condition will keep recurring. The eczema is a warning to Alan that he is pushing himself too hard. If he ignores this warning, he could find himself suffering from more serious effects of prolonged stress, such as high blood pressure or angina. His doctor has advised him to practice relaxation techniques to relieve the stress.

Action Plan

WORK
Try to negotiate a more reasonable workload. Excessive working hours and insufficient breaks will only cause a deterioration in work quality.

STRESS
To combat stress, make time for relaxation at the end of every working day.

DIET
Don't be tempted to skip meals. Always maintain a healthy, balanced diet, even if this means adapting mealtimes to fit around your busy working day.

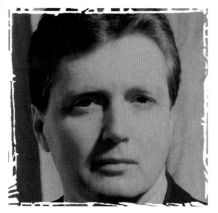

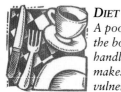

DIET
A poor diet reduces the body's ability to handle stress and makes it more vulnerable to illness.

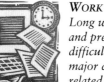

WORK
Long working hours and pressure to meet difficult targets are major causes of work-related stress.

STRESS
Previous sufferers of eczema often experience a recurrence during times of prolonged stress.

HOW THINGS TURNED OUT FOR ALAN

Alan discussed the problem of his workload with his manager and managed to negotiate some part-time assistance. Alan also began taking his lunch to work so he can take a quick break and eat healthfully without too much disruption of his work. Alan now sets aside one night a week for a cooking class. He enjoys the social interaction, and the results encourage him to eat properly. His eczema is finally starting to clear up.

DID YOU KNOW?
Some over-the-counter medications affect mood and emotional stability. Many cough and cold remedies, for example, contain ephedrine, which can cause nervousness and insomnia, and others may contain diphenhydramine, which has been known to bring on drowsiness.

relieve any physical stress that has built up during the day but also help your body to repair itself, and they increase your overall resistance to stress. Your mind benefits because the electrical activity in your brain slows down, making you feel calmer and more in control. Many people find that their memory and ability to concentrate improve as the mind feels less cluttered and overwhelmed. If you can distance yourself from problems and anxieties for a time, it may become possible to approach them from a new and more rational perspective.

GETTING ENOUGH SLEEP

Sleeping well is vital to feeling fresh and enthusiastic the following day. An occasional sleepless night can take its toll on energy levels, though it shouldn't have any long-lasting effect on general well-being. However, a prolonged period of sleeplessness can cause chronic fatigue and irritability, reducing the ability to concentrate and making the ups

and downs of life more difficult to bear. If you are having trouble getting to sleep, there are some simple steps you can take that may alleviate the problem. First, make sure that your bed is comfortable, with a mattress that supports your spine properly. Having a bedroom that is quiet, dark, and well ventilated will help too, as will setting a routine. During the day, get plenty of exercise and resist any temptation to take a nap. Avoid heavy meals late in the evening and keep away from caffeine and nicotine, both of which increase alertness. It's a good idea to unwind for an hour before going to bed by listening to music, watching television, or reading a book.

MAKING TIME FOR YOURSELF

If you spend the largest part of your time doing things for other people, such as working for your employer or looking after the needs of your family, it's important to take some time out just for yourself. How you spend this time—socializing, participating in sports, working on hobbies, going shopping for pleasure rather than necessity, or simply doing nothing in particular—is entirely up to you, as long as the activity is just for your own enjoyment.

Spending time on yourself makes you feel good because it allows you to escape from the stresses of life. It can also help raise your self-esteem. Taking the time and trouble to cater to your own needs demonstrates both

PLANNING YOUR TIME

Using time efficiently makes daily activity more productive and reduces frustration and stress. The following are a few tips for getting the most out of your day:

► *List priorities and estimate how long they will take. Be realistic in your judgment and don't set targets that are not feasible.*

► *Avoid procrastination; in particular, don't put off difficult jobs—they won't be any easier tomorrow. It is much more rewarding to get them out of the way; not only will you feel satisfaction, but you can then get on with enjoying the rest of the day.*

► *Always try to set aside some time for yourself. Take proper lunch breaks during your working days and spend a little time relaxing and enjoying yourself in the evenings and on the weekends.*

► *Establish routines to ensure that chores get done but do not let them become too rigid. Be flexible enough so that an interruption in your routine does not become a source of irritation.*

A SIMPLE RELAXATION TECHNIQUE

Practice this technique as a simple way to unwind each day. Lie on your back with your legs extended and your arms comfortably resting at your sides. Breathe in and out deeply and slowly a few times, then gently stretch the muscles in your toes and feet. As you relax them again, imagine them becoming increasingly heavy. Gradually move up your body, stretching and relaxing the muscles in your legs, pelvis, waist, hands and arms, chest, and finally your neck and head, until your whole body feels heavy and immobile on the floor. Enjoy this complete sense of relaxed heaviness, with the floor supporting your entire weight, for as long as you can without interruption.

A hard surface is best for this exercise, but you may want to cushion the head.

SIMPLE RELAXATION
Progressively stretching and relaxing each muscle is a good way to relax.

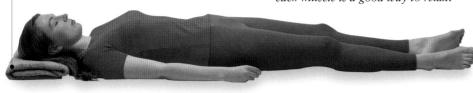

BEING SUPPORTIVE

To receive the benefits from a good network of friends, you also need to provide support and strength to others. Psychologist Stevan Hobfell has noted particular behaviors and attitudes in people who help friends and family to deal with stress. He claims that you are supportive if you

▶ are a good listener, show concern and interest, and are prepared to give time and attention to helping.

▶ express understanding of the other person's situation without claiming to have experienced identical distress.

▶ show affection for the person. Even a simple hug or pat on the arm can demonstrate your concern and interest.

SHARING YOUR FEELINGS
Being a good friend means being attentive and caring. It is important both to receive and to provide loving support.

to yourself and others that you as an individual are important. It is intriguing how often some people lose sight of their real interests and personalities as commitments to family, work, and social life start to take over. Thinking about who you are and what you really want can help you achieve a unique sense of completeness.

Expressing your thoughts openly can be difficult, however. Experiments have shown that fewer than 30 percent of people are willing to assert their ideas if these appear to run counter to or are vastly different from those of the majority. Even when individuals feel absolutely convinced that they are right, most are still too hesitant and doubtful to assert themselves. Many of the world's greatest politicians, philosophers, scientists, writers, and artists achieved renown through their unique expression of individuality and confident self-belief. People like Albert Einstein, Charles Darwin, and Martin Luther King all overcame public disapproval to become admired individuals and inspiring leaders in their fields.

ESTABLISHING A SUPPORT NETWORK

Regular social contact with other people is an important ingredient of emotional health and stability. This is particularly true for people who live alone, but even those in happy and loving relationships often need further stimulation. Friends are especially important because they provide an interest beyond the immediate family or workplace. They are an invaluable source of independent and objective advice, listening to your problems and offering companionship.

Much of the good feeling that derives from friendships comes from the sense of belonging and worth that they bring. The enjoyment of participating in events with others and feeling valued by them improves self-esteem and mental health. Friendships can also promote physical health because contentment keeps the body's immune system functioning properly.

It is rewarding to work hard at maintaining existing friendships and developing new ones and keeping in touch on a regular basis. The input of different opinions and feelings are a vital ingredient in achieving a healthy, balanced, and positive view of both ourselves and the outside world.

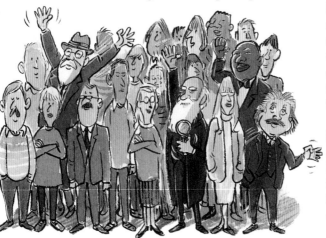

STANDING OUT IN A CROWD
Many famous people have fought against skepticism and disapproval to become great figures in their fields.

INDEX

159

ACKNOWLEDGMENTS

Carroll & Brown Limited
would like to thank
Lisa Jenson,
The Quindo Centre

Editorial assistance
Denise Alexander
Richard Emerson
Jennifer Mussett
Nadia Silver

Design assistance
Mercedes Pearson

DTP design
Elisa Merino

Photographic assistant
Alex Franklin
Mark Langridge

Picture research
Sandra Schneider

Photograph sources
8 AKG London
9 Nancy Kedersha,
  Science Photo Library
10 Popperfoto/Reuter
17 Wellcome Department of
  Cognitive Neurology, Science
  Photo Library
19 Tony Stone Images, David Tack
20 Collections, V.I.
21 The Ronald Grant Archive
22 The Ronald Grant Archive,
  copyright King Features Syndicate
23 The Maudsley Institute of
  Psychiatry
25 David McCarthy,
  The School of Pharmacy, London
26 Hulton Getty
27 (Top) National Library of
  Medicine, Science Photo Library
  (Bottom) Science Photo Library
28 Corbis-Bettman
29 Jules Selmes

32 (Top) Vincent Oliver,
  Science Photo Library
  (Bottom) Tony Stone Images,
  Penny Gentieu
37 (Left) Mary Evans Picture
  Library, Sigmund Freud
  copyright
  (Right) The Wellcome
  Institute Library, London
38 Galleria dell' Accademia,
  Florence, The Bridgeman
  Art Library
40 Rex Features
42 The Stock Market
44 Pictorial Press
46 The Stock Market
48 Rex Features
52 The Stock Market
54 The Stock Market
61 Aaron T. Beck
63 Archives of the History of
  American Psychology,
  University of Akron
98 Mary Evans Picture Library
102 Tony Stone Images
103 Musee d'Orsay, Paris, Peter
  Willi, Bridgeman Art Library
104 BSIP VEM, Science Photo
  Library
106 Jim Holmes, Axiom
109 (Top) Aviation Images,
  Mark Wagner
  (Bottom) NASA/Science Photo
  Library
110 Rex Features
112 (Top) Alan Benainous,
  Frank Spooner Pictures
  (Bottom) Liason, Frank Spooner
  Pictures
115 The Kobal Collection
116 The Ronald Grant Archive
118 Angela Hampton, Family Life
  Pictures
121 Corbis-Bettman
122 Mary Evans Picture Library/
  Sigmund Freud copyright
127 Corbis-Bettman
128 Corbis-Bettman

131 Science Museum, Science &
  Society Picture Library
132 Corbis-Bettman
134 The Quindo Centre
136 Mary Evans Picture Library
138 Corbis-Bettmann/UPI
140 AKG London
145 Ancient Art and Architecture
  Collections
146 (Top) Images Colour Library
  (Bottom) The Trustees of the
  British Museum
148 Jim Holmes, Axiom
150 Popperfoto

Illustrators
Melanie Barnes
George Foster
Rosamund Fowler
John Geary
Anni Jenkins
Joanna Venus
Anthea Whitworth
Angela Wood

Hair and make-up
Bettina Graham
Kim Menzies
Jessamina Owens

075–013-02